SURVIVING PA SCHOOL

CME4LIFE Presents:

SURVIVING PA SCHOOL

By John Bielinski, Jr.

Writers of the Round Table Press
PO Box 511, Highland Park, IL 60035
www.roundtablecompanies.com

Publisher: **Corey Michael Blake**
President: **Kristin Westberg**
Executive Editor: **Sarah Morrison**
Cover Designer: **Christy Bui**
Interior Designers: **Christy Bui, Sunny DiMartino**
Facts Keeper: **Mike Winicour**
Proofreader: **Adam Lawrence**
Last Looks: **Carly Cohen**
Project Manager: **Leeann Sanders**
Print and Digital Post Production: **Sunny DiMartino**

Printed in the United States of America

First Edition: March 2017
10 9 8 7 6 5 4 3 2 1

Library of Congress Cataloging-in-Publication Data
Bielinski, Jr., John.
Surviving pa school: secrets you must unlock to excel as a
physician assistant student / John Bielinski, Jr.—1st ed. p. cm.
ISBN Paperback: 978-1-939418-94-4
ISBN Digital: 978-1-939418-95-1
Library of Congress Control Number: 2017935793

RTC Publishing is an imprint of Writers of the Round Table, Inc.
Writers of the Round Table Press and the RTC Publishing logo
are trademarks of Writers of the Round Table, Inc.

I dedicate this book to the PA student. Yes, you.
The student who stays up late, who drinks knowledge
from a fire hose, and who is inspired to learn.

Contents

Foreword

It seems like I have known the author for a long time, but we first met in June of 2015 when he visited my home in Wake Forest, North Carolina. Although I am old enough to be his father, our relationship is more like that of two close brothers. It only took a few minutes for me to be engulfed by his enthusiasm for the PA profession. John is both knowledgeable and personable. We share many of the same hopes and dreams and respect for military veterans.

Since this is a book by a PA and for PAs, I would be remiss if I did not include a few words about my mentor and the founder of our profession, Eugene A. Stead, Jr. Dr. Stead was an extraordinary scientist, physician, teacher, and administrator. He was highly respected and admired, dedicated, and selfless. He had a unique ability to state complicated concepts in simple, witty language. Dr. Stead passed away in 2005 at the age of 96.

You are about to read a book chock-full of practical advice. If you will read and heed, you will become an integral part of the healthcare team. You and others like you will make it possible for many more people to receive the healthcare they need at a more affordable cost. You will be a physician's assistant! Resist becoming so busy that you do not have time to be a good listener. Listening lets the patient know you care—and you might learn something, too.

Ken Ferrell, PA
Duke University PA Program, Class of 1967

Acknowledgments

I want to acknowledge my wife, Michelle—a PA whom I met in PA school at King's College—for tolerating my forever ambition to grind.

I want to thank my kids, Johnny, Matthew, and Sarah, for being good kids that I am proud of. Remember, clean your rooms and set high goals.

I want to thank the North Carolina Academy of Physician Assistants for their continued support over the years and for having the absolute *best* CME conference in Myrtle Beach (www.ncapa.org).

Dwayne Williams: Thank you for your friendship and support. Your review book, *PANCE Prep Pearls*, remains my most recommended. Your passion in education is contagious (www.pancepreppearls.com).

Thanks also to Jennifer Carlquist, a truly gifted cardiology educator and artist. You are an educational catalyst—no one teaches about Brugada better.

I want to thank Scarlett and Joel Holcombe from Medical Mission Teams for introducing me to mission work (www.medicalmissionteams.org).

Thank you to Christina Beards, Frank Ambriz, Krisi Gindlesperger, and Mike Sharma.

Thank you to the many universities that have allowed me to speak to their students:

D'Youville College
Daemen College

Gannon University

Methodist University

Campbell University

University of Charleston

University of Texas Rio Grande Valley

University of Mount Union

Bay Path University

McMaster University

Pennsylvania College of Technology

King's College

Howard University

George Washington University

University of Maryland Eastern Shore

University of Maryland

Christian Brothers University

Bethel University

University of the Cumberlands

Marshall B. Ketchum University

Jefferson University

Mercer University

East Carolina University

Finally, many thanks to the people who have contributed information to this book:

Ruth Ballweg, MPA, PA
Professor Emeritus
Department of Family Medicine
School of Medicine
University of Washington

Wallace Boeve, EdD, PA-C
Program Director
Physician Assistant Program
Bethel University

Christopher Hanifin, PA-C
Chair, Department of Physician Assistant
School of Health and Medical Sciences
Seton Hall University

Henry H. Heard, DHSc, PA-C
Clinical Assistant Professor
College of Health Professions
Physician Assistant Program

Jocelyn Hook, MPAS, PA-C
Clinical Coordinator, Clinical Professor
King's College Department of PA Studies

Nancy Hurwitz, PA-C MHP
Director of Clinical Education
MCPHS University PA Program, Boston

James Kilgore, PhD, PA-C, DFAAPA
Director/Assistant Professor
Physician Assistant Program
Department of Clinical and Diagnostic Sciences
School of Health Professions
Associate Scientist
UAB Center for Exercise Medicine
University of Alabama at Birmingham

Richard E. Murphy, PA-C, MBA, DFAAPA
Director, Physician Assistant Program
Associate Professor of Surgery, Public Health and
    Community Medicine
Tufts University School of Medicine

Robert Philpot, PhD, PA-C, DFAAPA
Professor and Chairman
Department of Physician Assistant Studies
Mississippi College

Deborah Summers, M.S., PA-C
Assistant Professor and Clinical Education Coordinator
Graduate Professional Physician Assistant Program
University of the Sciences

Kristin Thomson, MHS, PA-C
Director, Associate Professor
Touro Physician Assistant Program (Manhattan Campus)

Gary B. Tooley, DHSc, PA-C, DFAAPA
COL (ret) USA
Associate Professor/Director of Academics
Christian Brothers University PA Program

Gerald R. Weniger, MEd, MPAS, ATC, PA-C
Program Director and Assistant Professor
James Madison University PA Program

Maddie Windstein, PA-C
Physician Assistant in Emergency Medicine
Our Lady of the Lake Regional Medical Center
Baton Rouge, Louisiana

Introduction

My name is John Bielinski, Jr. I'm a physician assistant (PA), teacher, lecturer, and founder of CME4LIFE, a company that takes a unique, accessible approach to teaching continuing medical education. I'm honored that you chose to use this book as a guide to help you through your PA studies. As a career PA and an international lecturer on PA studies, I've learned a great many things that I want to share with you. Over the past twenty years, I've taught emergency medicine and other board review topics at twenty-five PA schools; colleges hire me to come in and train their PA students on how to pass their board exams.

Often, I think: *I wish I'd had the opportunity to work with these students from the beginning—we could have avoided so many of these problems.* Good habits need to start early, and I feel that students can benefit tremendously from learning the ins and outs of studying, playing PA school politics, and practicing medicine from the very beginning.

I went to King's College in Wilkes-Barre, Pennsylvania, and I graduated in 1997. I wish I could tell you I was so smart; I wish I could tell you I became a PA because I observed trends in medicine; I wish I could tell you I selected that particular PA program because I was wise. To be very honest, I got really lucky. I was a student with struggles—my grades were so bad that I didn't graduate high school on time. I joined and served in the Marines, and my military background likely played a large part in my being accepted to PA school. Since then, though, I've gained a lot of wisdom about what it takes to flourish as a PA student and as a working PA. I've been in staff meetings to discuss struggling students. I've spoken with teachers about the disconnect between curricula and testing. I've spoken with thousands of students about the challenges they are facing.

I love being a PA. I love teaching, and I love helping patients. I love the education process. I love the trials and tribulations of my work, and I love being around my colleagues. But being a PA is very hard, and PA school is borderline overwhelming.

Different PA schools have very different cultures when it comes to how to behave and what is acceptable. But one thing they all have in common is that they really need you to pass your boards. There is tremendous political pressure on a PA program to have high pass rates on the boards—not just pressure from the academic institution itself, but also pressure from the governing body that approves of PA programs, the Accreditation Review Commission on Education for the Physician Assistant (ARC-PA). If a program's boards pass rates are low, then all sorts of restrictions are placed on the program. So PA schools have different ways of ensuring high pass rates. Some PA schools will nurture you through any difficulties you may be having. The hardest part was getting in, but now that you're in, as long as you don't quit they'll get you through. But not all PA schools are like that. With some PA schools, if you don't make high enough grades, you get one warning and then you get kicked out.

This is the biggest landmine you want to avoid in PA school: getting kicked out or decelerated. But PA school involves many other landmines at various stages in the game that can be devastating. The intense studying, the political aspects, and the need to study for the long term are all areas of PA school that you will need to understand and navigate, using this book as your roadmap.

Regardless of what kind of program you are in, this book will help you be a better PA student in your first year during the didactic phase, help you be a better PA student in your second year during rotations, help you pass your boards, and help you be a better PA someday.

Overview of Contents

First off, I'll give you the rundown on what you need to know and do before you even arrive at PA school. You may be surprised by how big this section is; I'm going to really delve deeply into how to position yourself even before PA school, because as with most things in life, preparation is the key to success. You can prevent a lot of problems by gaining the right tools and mindset from the beginning. Setting this groundwork will be incredibly valuable down the line.

Then I'll give you an overview of the major landmines of your didactic phase, as well as guidance on how to avoid them. The didactic phase of PA school—your first year, made up of traditional academic classes—is like studying for a big final exam, but for a whole year straight. For the entire year, you spend eight hours a day in class, and then you go home and still have four or six hours of studying left—and that lasts for two semesters. It is almost like you're learning four years of medical school content in one year. I'll show you how to study the material, move to the next level, and not get overwhelmed. I will give you the scoop, the pearls, and the tools for keeping up academically.

Next, I'll guide you through your rotations, your second year of PA school, where you spend three- or four-week cycles in various healthcare facilities in order to gain hands-on experience. A good student who can really get the most out of rotations will be five times further ahead than a student who passively goes through rotations. As a long-time preceptor myself—I was honored to win the Preceptor of the Year Award from the Rochester Institute of Technology PA program in 2002—I have the insider's scoop on how to get the most out of your rotations. You'll learn how to develop a deep knowledge base and interact effectively with patients, while also learning the political elements of working with doctors, nurses, and ancillary staff.

After that, I'll take you through the next phase—preparing for your Physician Assistant National Certifying Exam (PANCE). Over the last three years, that's really been my passion and calling: teaching PA board preparation. The bottom line is, ladies and gentlemen, this has to start right away. I'm going to teach you, with this book, how to start preparing for your boards right from the get-go.

How to Use This Book

I encourage you to read this book all the way through before you arrive at PA school, and then I recommend that you return to it often. Make notes about parts that especially apply to your situation. When you're at different stages of your education, different parts of the book will resonate more with you. The main thing to keep in mind is that when it comes to a lot of the concepts we'll talk about—studying for the long term, for example, as well as playing politics in PA school—you'll want to have a solid understanding of the factors at work before even beginning, because you're going to want to lay your foundation early.

A Note on My Recommendations and Resources

Throughout this book, I make various recommendations and judgments about resources and strategies that may prove helpful to you. Please understand that my opinions are mine and mine alone—but I have earned those opinions through decades as a career PA, classroom instructor, preceptor, and board review lecturer. My only aim in making recommendations is to help you succeed, and I have done my best to be completely transparent and honest in my advice.

Chapter 1
So, You're Going to Be a PA Student

"PA school is not for the less-than-dedicated, faint of heart, or shy!"
—Dr. James Kilgore

You've Made a Great Choice!

The health landscape is great for PAs. Here's the deal—when you look at the cost of healthcare in the United States, coupled with inflation, there's no question that our system is going bankrupt, and to fix it there needs to be sweeping reform. The good news for you is that PAs are the solution. PA schools are popping up left and right, because not only do PAs save money, but we also help a ton of people. A medical practice that employs three physicians could very easily get rid of two of them and hire four PAs instead. In doing so, the medical practice would make money and have increased capacity to care for more patients. The PA model of care is successful, and relying more heavily on PAs is a strong trend globally.

You'll have financial security. When you graduate from PA school, you will be in the upper middle class, based on income, for the rest of your life. If you invest wisely, you'll retire as a multimillionaire. That's the financial side of it, and there's no reason to think that this trend won't continue.

You'll have wonderful job mobility. As a PA, you will have extreme lateral mobility. This kind of lateral mobility means that as PAs, we can jump medical specialties at any time. In my career, I have always worked in the field of emergency medicine, yet at any time, I could say, "I have decided to go into cardiology." I could go into gastroenterology or even nephrology. I could change roles, and this would not require any official change in my license. That's not the case with physicians or nurse practitioners.

PAs also have a significant degree of vertical mobility. I know a number of PAs who, like myself, are in the position to run emergency rooms, where we take care of patients in cardiac arrest, deliver babies, and deal with major trauma. Again, there is no reason to think that this kind of job mobility will not continue; based on what I know from speaking with the governing bodies at the National Commission for the Certification of Physician Assistants (NCCPA), lateral and vertical mobility for PAs will be preserved at all costs.

You can be somebody's miracle. I remember when I got my acceptance letter to King's College. I was in my kitchen, and when I opened the letter and saw "Congratulations" at the top of the paper, I jumped up and down and cried. Since then I've heard from many students about their reactions to the phone calls, emails, and letters they received telling them that they were going to be PA students. Many of these students tell me that they cried, something that always impresses me—it's clear how passionate we are about what we do. Being a PA is an absolutely wonderful calling that I'm deeply proud to be a part of.

Of course, you will face challenges—whether as a student or once you're out in the workforce—and at those times, you need to cling to your life raft, the true *why* of medicine, which is that you have the capability to be somebody's miracle. Remember that *you* have the ability to help a patient control his cholesterol, or finally stop smoking, or finally agree to get a polyp removed before it becomes metastatic brain cancer.

Will you be someone's miracle? The answer is yes—more than you will ever know. You will become uniquely qualified to care for people when they're at their sickest, most desperate, and most concerned. You will be in a position to prevent disease, diagnose illnesses, and treat people. You will gain patients' confidence to the extent that they will tell you things they would not tell their priest or their spouse.

You will break the news of cancer to a patient, but you will also provide families news that surgeries were successful. I cannot tell you how many patients I have pronounced dead in my career—but I also cannot tell you how many times I've resuscitated critically ill patients.

You knew there were other choices in medicine; you could have become a nurse, a paramedic, or a physician. All of those professions have their own advantages and disadvantages, yet you decided to become a PA.

We make a good living and have a good life. I really want to welcome you to this profession.

What to Consider if You're Still Choosing a School

Schools are very different and have very different environments. PA schools are different. There are regional differences in PA schools, and there are cultural differences in PA schools. In some programs, the guys all wear ties; in other programs, most students wear running clothes to class.

Some PA schools are incredibly nurturing, holding the basic philosophy that as long as you don't quit, you will be remediated until you succeed. This was the case at King's College—they made it very clear to me that as long as I kept working, they were going to get me through PA school. When I got into my program, I was scared. I felt like an impostor, to be quite honest with you. I felt it was just a matter of time before I got weeded out. But then I saw that the program would support me as long as I kept on working, and that love and nurturing were really important to me.

The first part-time faculty position I took at a college in Buffalo, New York, had the exact opposite approach. If you failed a course, you immediately went to academic suspension and then deceleration. If you failed a course, they would drop you very quickly. It was cutthroat and merciless. I remember being in faculty meetings discussing this approach. Those in charge were very black-and-white about it—if you failed a course, you were pushed back, and there was nothing you could do about it short of taking legal action.

Think hard about which kind of program you will flourish in, and do your homework about the programs you're applying to. Try to speak or email with current students to determine what the culture in a given school is like.

*"As someone who travels around to many programs—
both domestically and internationally—I see many
errors in lumping PA programs together when in fact
each is its own culture. Some research is important
for candidates to figure out where they best fit in
terms of values, goals, and past experience."*
—Ruth Ballweg

Faculty is an important consideration. I think the staff is
the biggest determining factor of a good PA school. Some
of the most senior PA schools where I've taught have had
excessive staff turnover for one reason or another. When
that happens, you're getting a bunch of wildcard instructors.
I'd rather have a PA school that's been around five years
and had a stable core faculty for those five years than
a PA program that's been around for thirty years but keeps
having staff turnover. In the latter case, you never quite
know what you're going to get.

I'm a martial artist, and it's the same with martial arts
schools. If I go into a black belt class, and all the students
got their black belts at that school, it tells me a lot. It tells
me that the school has been around for a long time and
has retained membership for a long time.

This is another area where you can do your due
diligence: researching faculty and perhaps asking some
current students about their thoughts and experiences.

Take finances into account. Most PA students finish PA
school with some amount of debt from student loans. This
shouldn't frighten you. However, finances will definitely be
a consideration for many students. Do your research about
what various PA schools will cost you, what your loans will

look like, what the job landscape in that area will look like for PAs, and so forth.

Get Into the Right Mindset

Start with the why. As a PA, you'll face long nights of studying, long nights of being at the hospital, long drives, difficult nursing staff, and tricky patients. During these tough times, you're going to need to have strong, internalized, focused motivation. What's driving you? What's the fire inside of you? What truly is your motivation for becoming a PA?

There are many different motivations, some of them better than others. Some people just want to work in healthcare. Some people want the money or the job security. None of these reasons are wrong. But a deeper *why* is going to make you study longer, wake up earlier, and try harder. That's really important.

I encourage you to create a mission statement that is highly personal. You can refer to it as motivation, and you can add to it and evolve it as you evolve in your education and in your profession. In my personal mission statement, I included that I deeply want to help people. I deeply want to have the answers when people are sick, and I want to be that person in an intense situation who either has the right answers or is able to guide patients appropriately. My mission has always driven me to emergency medicine or critical care.

Where will your mission guide you?

"Maintaining energy and enthusiasm becomes increasingly more difficult as time goes on, but it can be done. Remember WHY you want to be a PA, and never let that go."
—Deborah Summers

There's no whining in PA school. I believe that no PA school is perfect. But please remember, there is no whining. Do not start complaining. You're going to have classmates who bother you a little bit. You don't whine. There will be instructors who teach you conflicting information. You don't whine. You're going to feel ill-prepared for some tests; no whining. There's a time and a place to have professional conversations about concerns, but whining has no place, from day one until your final day.

If you are someone who complains a lot, your complaining is really a prediction of how you're going to perform professionally. In your career, there will be conflicts. There will be concerns. But throughout, your human interaction skills need to be optimal; medicine is at its core a field of human interaction. PA school will be difficult, but you need to be incredibly mature and incredibly professional, no exceptions.

Understand that your teachers want to help you. In PA school, you will have base instructors and adjunct faculty members. Your base instructors are the people you see regularly, typically full-time faculty members. Most of them are PAs, though you will also likely have some physicians on staff.

Some of your instructors will be uniquely qualified in the topics they're teaching. Ideally, you'll have a PA with twenty years of clinical experience in cardiology teaching you about electrocardiograms (EKGs). That's your best instructor: someone who's been there and done that clinically, but who also has textbook knowledge. Unfortunately, a lot of instructors are asked to teach on topics they have not practiced clinically. I see this often when it comes to teaching blood gases and EKGs. You're going to know very quickly who knows what she's talking about, and who is just teaching from a book. Here's where you have to be realistic, kind, and forgiving. Be kind to your instructors, and know that they're doing their best to teach you the concepts.

I have met scores of PA school faculty members, and I will absolutely guarantee you something. They are not there for the money. They are making approximately $20,000 less than they could be if they were working clinically. They are teaching because they want you to be successful—but your success does not depend on your instructors. It is the student's responsibility to learn.

If you have an EKG instructor who is not able to communicate or test effectively, or if you have a faculty member struggling to teach acid base in a way that makes sense, guess what? It's your job to go learn it anyway. You learn it from a textbook. You learn it from Wikipedia or Medscape. You find some online resource or book you can learn it from. We are in a tremendous video culture, where you can look up almost anything on YouTube. It's your job as a student to learn. Remember, there's no whining in PA school.

Maintain an internal locus of control. A concept related to these other issues—avoiding whining, as well as taking responsibility for your own learning—is *locus of control*, a concept developed by Julian B. Rotter. If you have an external locus of control, you believe that things happen to you without your being able to impact the situation. If you have an internal locus of control, however, you understand that you have agency over situations or at the very least how you respond to them. Those with an external locus of control are reactive, whereas those with an internal locus of control are proactive. Proactive people make things happen. They get things done. They take charge of their own education and careers. You need to understand that you are in control of your decisions; you are in control of your life.

Avoid comparisons and focus on development.
PA school is no different than any other academic environment in which most people believe that if you get an A, or if you get 100 percent, then you are smart, you get the star, you get the cookie, you get the accolades, and your report card goes on the fridge. We have been trained from a very young age to produce the grades, and thus there is a natural tendency for competition when it comes to grades.

When you go through PA school, you will need to have *knowledge* that enables you to help people when they are sick. As a faculty member, it used to drive me crazy when someone would raise his or her hand and ask whether something was going to be on a test. When all you are doing is dancing for the grade, you're losing sight of the point, which is to become a better clinician.

What you need to understand is that it is not about you anymore. When you become a PA and you get your license, you have to surrender yourself for your patients' best interests; you have to do what is right for your patients and not for yourself. This selflessness needs to begin with how you approach your grades. PA school is not about your grades or your ego or whether you were valedictorian, because none of your patients will care about that—they will want to feel supported and guided and well taken care of. Nobody looking at your resume cares about your grades, either. They care about whether you're going to fit into the culture of the team and whether you have the required knowledge to do the job.

In PA school, it is very important to focus on what you really need to learn in order to ensure that a) you don't fail out and b) you are really learning how to help others. So, of course grades matter to some extent, because they serve as one measure of learning. But I encourage you to focus on them as just that: *one* measure of learning. I encourage you to work hard and get the grades you need, but even more than that, to get the *knowledge* you need.

When I was in PA school, I worked very hard on the hardcore medical classes. I busted my butt on GI, gastroenterology, pulmonary, and cardiac. We also had a course in genetics and an epidemiology course, but I knew I wouldn't fail out of the program, so I didn't put one ounce of effort into those classes. I focused on the things that really put me in a good position to help my future patients. I deemphasized what were for me the unimportant classes, and I really emphasized the classes that would help me get ahead. The grade was not what was important.

Of course, your situation may be very different; if you are in a very strict program, you may need to focus on keeping your grades high in order to avoid being decelerated. My point is that you should not confuse good grades with the kind of deep knowledge that enables you to be an effective clinician, which is most important.

Understand the difference between natural and social learning. When it comes to learning, you have a social system and a natural system. The elements of a social system relate to how people quantify and manipulate knowledge. Traditional test taking relies heavily on factors like memorizing terms, selecting the right answer from a set, and putting information in a certain order. The fact that you got into PA school in the first place means you are likely skilled when it comes to these kinds of social factors—you can probably cram for a test and get a good grade.

The elements of a natural system, on the other hand, entail a much wider range of factors that have to do with real people and situations. In a natural system, you are taking in everything you see, hear, taste, smell, and feel and translating that into information and knowledge that inform your decisions. Social systems are more black-and-white, whereas natural systems are often gray. Social systems are controlled; natural systems are chaotic.

The danger comes in assuming that because you are knowledgeable on these social scales, you are automatically capable in natural settings. If you get an A on a test about infectious diseases, you may think you understand infectious diseases and are able to diagnose and treat them—but that's not accurate. In Driver's Ed, you take a written test, which is a social system test—but you also need to actually get out there on the road, in a natural system, to show that you can put all of your memorized facts into kinesthetic practice. You can memorize a book about farming, showing skill in social systems, but what will actually matter when it comes to your success as a farmer is developing skills in the natural system—gauging how your crops respond to different soil pH, getting the amount of water to the right level, and dealing with any pests that come your way.

True medicine is a natural system. True medicine isn't multiple-choice. You need to develop your knowledge and experience in order to gain a deeper understanding of the factors at play and possible courses of action. As with farming, you have to consistently put in time, effort, and resources to have a fertile harvest.

Of course, PA school involves a lot of social learning, particularly during your didactic year. You will learn how your instructors test, and you will figure out what kinds of memorization and manipulation of information are required in order to get the grades you need. But because medicine is such a natural system, those who create the PANCE— the board exam—design the exam questions to require an incredibly deep and layered understanding of medicine. As you will see in chapter 4, which addresses the PANCE, there are definitely social elements of the exam. However, social learning alone—that is, cramming like you are probably used to doing for tests—will not be sufficient to pass your boards, because they aim to test you on the intricate, more chaotic level of a natural system. By the time I'm having this conversation with most students, they're getting ready for the boards and they're about 80–90 percent through with their rotations. Already the cow is out of the barn if you have not been studying for your boards all along.

Make Sure You Have What You Need

You know that you have a period of time before you start your education in PA school. Most of us find out early, and then we have three, four, or even five months until we start. If you're like me, you are an overachiever, and you really want to be adequately prepared for when you walk in the door. Some schools will have an agenda for what they want you to study before you walk in on day one—if that's the case with your program, that's wonderful. But a lot of schools don't. They just say, "We'll see you on the first day." Guys, that's unacceptable!

You are going into a profession in which you need to deeply know concepts, and it's best to get started as early as you can.

Master your medical terminology. Before you arrive at PA school, you have to have a mastery of medical terminology. I recommend picking up *Medical Terminology for Health Professions*, 7th edition, by Ann Ehrlich. You need an absolute detailed mastery of the Latin that forms the basis for medical words. If not, you're going to be behind the eight ball. You need to either get a medical terminology review book or take an additional course.

If I say words like cholecystectomy and choledocholithiasis, you need to know what they mean; you need to have a visceral, automatic understanding of basic terminology, or else you're going to have a tough time keeping up with the instructors.

They're going to expect you to know things, and you won't want to be chasing your tail when it comes to understanding what they say in class or interpreting your notes.

Study up on pharmacology. Once you have an unbelievably high degree of understanding of medical terminology, you have to study pharmacology. Lecturing across the United States, I am constantly asking people, "What do you feel is weak about your program?" Almost every program I work with is weak on pharmacology. I know exactly why this happens. Pharmacology is a daunting, amazing topic and is typically taught by a pharmacist rather than by a clinician. When you have a pharmacist teaching PAs, a tremendous amount of information is lost in translation. A pharmacist may know fancy stuff that looks really good to the governing body, but to my mind, clinicians are in a better position to teach other clinicians. Clinicians may not know all the science of an antibiotic, but they understand the clinical application of that antibiotic much better—when to use it, and when not to use it.

In order to fill potential gaps in your pharmacology education, my advice is to get a basic book on mechanisms of actions of pharmacology. I recommend *Pharmacology*, 3rd edition (Lippincott's Illustrated Review Series), by Howland, Mycek, Harvey, and Champe. Work on some key topics, such as the sympathetic and parasympathetic nervous systems. You need to know about the cardiac medicines, like a beta blocker, a calcium channel blocker, an ACE inhibitor, and digoxin.

Buy your books. As with any college class, you will be assigned a list of books that you have to buy. Some books are going to be wonderful resources for you, and some books are more designed as reference books to be used on an as-needed basis. What happens is that faculty members are compelled to include a reference text in their book list; this makes their course look authentic and legitimate. When I taught laboratory medicine, I needed to put a lab medicine book on my syllabus, although I was teaching pretty much right from my notes. If it was up to me, I wouldn't have required a book, but the program I was teaching for insisted that I include a text.

Students quickly realize which books are useful learning tools and which books are extraneous. Those extraneous books spend a lot of time on the shelf. Yet it's very difficult to know in advance which faculty members are going to use the books on their syllabi, and which are not. This may be information you can get from your senior classmates. In any case, my advice is to buy the books— buying used online or from senior classmates is fine— unless you get pretty conclusive information saying that you will not need a book.

One of the things that PA students need to put a lot of time into is EKG interpretation. There is a book called *Rapid Interpretation of EKG's* by Dale Dubin. It is a very old book that is time-tested, and you can progress in that book without needing an instructor. If you think you could benefit from some extra support in this area, I do recommend this book as a supplement to your learning and studying.

Get any other equipment you'll need. I advise getting an external audio recorder. It would be wonderful for you to get into the habit of recording lectures. This way, you get to listen to them repeatedly and pick up the finer points. I found this strategy really important in my own learning— I'm a real auditory learner. If your recordings are poor, you can just erase them, and there's no harm, no foul.

Also, an audio recorder gives you tremendous

resources in making use of all your time—you can listen to recordings of lectures on your commute, for example. I found this practice critically important, and I was a big fan of listening to lectures while in the car throughout my rotations and in fact throughout my first eighteen years as a PA. I still listen to audiobooks all the time, and I feel this habit has been the biggest part of my continual growth after PA school.

I also recommend a great external hard drive. You will need to save and back up a ton of information and resources.

When it comes to figuring out your housing, transportation, and other essentials, you are on your own. You're going to need a car, particularly in your second year, when you're traveling to different sites and locations.

A word on medical equipment: You will need to buy the necessary equipment: a stethoscope, an ophthalmoscope, an otoscope, and a tuning fork. What typically happens in PA programs is you come in and then an equipment rep will come right into the class, show you all the equipment, and hand out order sheets. Unless you can find these instruments somewhere cheaper, and you are certain they will still be reliable, I can't see much real value in buying this equipment before school begins. I would caution you that you don't need the super-expensive cardiology stethoscope; a run-of-the-mill stethoscope will be just fine. For a lot of the high-end stethoscopes, you need to have very sensitive ears even to detect much of a difference. I do recommend a long cord. If you have a really short cord, you will hear better, yes—but you are going to be really close to the patient and that can get a little bit uncomfortable at times.

Prepare for the PA School Lifestyle

You'll need exceptional time-management, scheduling, and planning skills. In PA school, you're going to have to have your own system of organization. You have to know exactly when assignments are due, and you have to really study the course syllabus.

Living by a schedule is very important when it comes to studying and keeping your eye on upcoming deliverables, tests, quizzes, and hand-in assignments. Every time you are given a task or deliverable, 100 percent of the time it must immediately go on your schedule. You may think you'll remember something without putting it on paper, or you may think you'll remember to put it on the schedule later, but if you're wrong it can cause a very regrettable situation. I think it's a really good plan to have one person in the class be the class secretary and use a community calendar to keep track of all the assignments and when they are due. If a paper is announced that is due next Friday, that person can immediately put it on the calendar, and everyone else can access it.

> *"Be organized! I used a calendar with vertical hourly times so I could fill in every bit of time with a specific designation (classes, tests, studying of each subject, appointments, eating, sleeping if there was any time left). This helped me to keep on track and not waste time between classes! Also, I love highlighters, so I would fill in the boxes with different colors based on the type of activity (class time, study time, quiz, test)."*
> —Maddie Windstein

Be a consummate professional. Ladies and gentlemen, you start building your reputation very early. The professors who teach you will most likely be the same ones who you'll eventually ask for references upon graduation—or they're going to know somebody in your local community who's going to want to hire you. Going through PA school is a maturing process. Once you get there, you need to represent yourself professionally from the very beginning and at all times.

This is the time to start practicing emotional intelligence and watching what you say to faculty members and student teachers. You need to talk to classmates in a professional manner. You need to talk to your professors in a professional manner. You don't send off emails or text messages that are not highly professional.

I cannot tell you how many jobs are made or broken by water cooler references. A big problem in PA school is when two different instructors come in and they bring different messages. So one instructor may say, "This is the antibiotic of choice for urinary tract infection," and another instructor may cite a different antibiotic. Some people will take a very immature approach and cause conflict about it in class: "Well, the other teacher says . . ." This creates problems. It is not professional.

You have to learn how to approach faculty members with political smarts, tact, and humility. Instead of pointing out a disparity, approach the situation from the perspective of having some confusion surrounding the topic. Position yourself as wanting to clear up your misunderstanding: "Would you please clarify this for me?" Egos can be very big in medicine, and if you get on somebody's bad side, it can come back to bite you, and I am speaking from personal experience. When it comes to the professional language you use—whether you are talking about the program, the faculty, or a test—you should always talk like the person you're talking about can hear you.

Being a PA means being the ultimate middleman. You ain't a doc, and you ain't a nurse—you are a middleman. You will be in the front row observing patients, and then you'll have to take that information from person to person. This means you have to be the ultimate communicator; some of the very best PAs I have ever worked with were restaurant servers who had developed extremely respectful and accurate communication skills. I encourage you to use PA school as a place to start learning how to communicate thoroughly and professionally.

> *"Professionalism starts on day one and never ends. This cannot be stressed enough. Never start an email, 'Hey professor X' or call your professor or preceptor by their first name unless asked to do so. Proper dress, hygiene, and courtesy to faculty, staff, and fellow students are of utmost importance. You are being evaluated every moment. Also, PA programs are graduate school—not college, not high school. You are an adult, so act like one. Faculty should NEVER hear from your parents, except in an emergency or at graduation."*
> —Deborah Summers

Handle your social media wisely. Professionalism includes not only your in-person conduct, but also your social media presence. If I know John Smith is coming to my ER for a month, that is a lot of time I am going to put into this guy's education, so I will check his Facebook, his Twitter, and his Instagram. Everybody does it. All your accounts need to be incredibly professional and clean. If I see pictures of John Smith drinking beers on a beach, looking all out of it, then he is coming into that rotation already with a strike against him. I encourage you to ensure that you would feel comfortable with any professional colleague seeing what you're putting out there online. You are a young student hungry to learn—you don't want anybody forming preconceived notions about you. My advice is to lock up your social media for friends only, make sure none of your pictures are shown, and have a LinkedIn account that is very professional. That is the right way to go.

Be proactive. I am going to say this very frankly: if you are a very shy person, you are going to need to stretch yourself in PA school and as a PA. If you are naturally timid, you are going to have a really tough time putting yourself out there in the didactic phase, you are going to have a really tough time getting the most out of rotations, and you are eventually going to struggle to connect with patients once you are a working PA.

If you are very passive and you have difficulty taking the reins, you are going to have a tremendously difficult time in medicine, which is a field based on interpersonal connection. In medicine, when you can get people to like you—not just patients, but also coworkers—your job is going to be easier. Medicine is an occupation of perception, meaning that the way patients perceive you as a medical provider has a great deal of bearing on how they contribute to the process and whether they follow your advice.

For example, if you are really timid and shy and feel uncomfortable asking people if you can join their study group, you are not going to be getting all you could from your PA school experience. I encourage you to remember that this is not about you anymore—it is about serving your future patients. I encourage you to stretch beyond your comfort zone a little bit and put yourself out there.

Know how to network. In addition to updating your LinkedIn page, I recommend that you reach out to your state organization—your state's branch of the American Academy of Physician Assistants (AAPA)—and join as a student member. This won't cost you much money or time, but it can go on your resume and will allow you to meet people, which is unbelievably powerful for long-term success. Most state organizations have student rates and will give you discounts on conferences (although I don't recommend going to conferences during your didactic phase). I am involved with a bunch of state organizations; while I'm at a meeting, if I have a student come up to me who just impresses me—someone who is hardworking and diligent, someone who is ready to take this profession by the horns—I am endeared to that student and I want to help that student, whether that means helping out with a job search or helping out when it comes to making additional contacts.

Most programs are pretty good at separating the senior class from the junior class. I know of very few programs that actually mingle the classes. My advice is that when you are in your didactic year, you talk to a senior classmate and say, "Can I ask you a favor that I promise I will pay forward?" In almost every instance, someone is going to say yes. Then you ask, "Do you mind if I get your phone number and email address so that if I have any problems or struggles or I need some advice, I can reach out to you?" Again, almost everyone will say yes to this kind of politely worded, reasonable request. My advice is not to have just one person, but to have two or three of them you reach out to at various times for some help. Say one particular teacher is tough; reach out to one of your senior contacts and say, "Can you give me some advice on how this teacher tests, how he looks at things, and how she grades?"

Your PA school instructors are going to have office hours, but if you take advantage of office hours, I would do it strategically and with intention. Too many times, people want to hobnob or just hang out. If you have a focused question because you are really missing a concept, that is one thing. But for the love of god, don't go into office hours with a question you could have spent five minutes going online to figure out, because it will only make you look lazy.

Plan to prioritize your health and well-being. I think it is really important to make sure you take the time to stay engaged and fresh in your studies, and that means devoting time to exercise, nutrition, relaxation, and spiritual connection. I think some people get so busy working that they forget what they need to stay sharp.

When I'm talking to a new PA class, one of the first things I say to the students is, "My expectation is that you are going to gain a student or two by the time the didactic phase is over," and people look at me like, "What are you talking about?" In my experience, everybody in class seems to gain about five or ten pounds, so if you weigh the whole class collectively at the beginning of that didactic phase and then again at the end, their weight will go up by about two hundred total pounds. So you don't want to gain another student. How will you avoid gaining weight? More broadly, how will you take care of your body?

I would answer with another question: When do your best ideas come to you? Whatever that looks like for you, make sure you do it. I think exercise is very important for any high achiever to involve in his or her routine. For you, this could mean going to play racquetball, it could mean going for a run, it could mean going to a yoga class or a martial arts class, or it could mean going to the gym and playing some music and pushing some weights around. Whatever you choose, it has got to be something that is built into your schedule.

If you can go play racquetball—or whatever your activity of choice happens to be—with someone who is in your study group, that is good for you. You can review concepts in a way that is engaging, and I have found that the best and quickest way to manage a squirrelly brain is exercise. You want to study harder? Make sure you are incorporating some exercise.

The other key is to be specific and goal-oriented. How are you staying physically healthy? A lot of people will say, "Well, I'm watching what I eat." What do you mean you are watching what you eat? "I try not to eat fast food." Well, that is not good enough for a high-functioning individual, which is what you are. You have to have a plan. How are you doing with drinking water? Keep a log. How are you doing with cutting back on simple carbohydrates? Track it. My advice is to drink a lot of water, get a lot of protein and vegetables, avoid processed foods, and avoid eating too many grains.

I encourage you to develop systems in order to ensure that you're taking care of yourself, whether that means an exercise routine, a nutrition tracking app, reminders on your phone to drink water—whatever works for you.

Plan to nurture your relationships. You need to spend time with your loved ones, and it has got to be dedicated quality time that is proactive rather than reactive. If you have a boyfriend, girlfriend, spouse, kids, or any combination of those, PA school is going to strain your relationships. It is not uncommon at all for marriages not to make it through PA school, because all of your time is dominated by class and studying. You come home to a spouse and kids who haven't seen you all day and are eager to spend time with you, but you are freaking out because you have a test tomorrow and you still have to study for at least four hours. What does this mean for you?

It means you've got to come home and make it a rule that you don't study for ninety minutes. Instead you spend time with the family. It means no phones, no TV. You are going to spend time with your girlfriend and your dog, whatever your situation looks like. Then, at the end of the ninety minutes, you go off into your study bubble, with strict boundaries and no interruptions.

This arrangement requires a high level of emotional maturity and discipline; you are going to need to keep your life in balance. You are going to come home, try to decompress, have a bite to eat, spend some quiet time with the people you love, and then go back to work. This system has to do with really clearly defining your boundaries and being very strict with your scheduling.

A word on finances and working: It is very rare these days that PAs go through school without student loans. I took out some student loans, and I also borrowed money from my family. It is important for you to set yourself up financially to where you do not have to work and you are not obligated to work, because quite frankly I think that is suicide. I believe that any amount of time you spend at a side job would be better spent studying. If you are making $10–$12 an hour working as a nurse's aid because you want to keep some money coming in, is that really worth it? If you have a job, and if—or more likely, when—you go south, and your grades go bad, you have no one to blame but yourself. You are not going to get any sympathy from anyone if you were working ten hours a week while going through PA school. Live off student loans. Live within your means. Don't take on any extra responsibilities.

Chapter 2

Your First Year: The Didactic Phase

"PA programs are roughly two years in length. To
cover the material, the typical PA student must be
prepared to drink knowledge from a six-inch high-
pressure hose twenty-four hours per day from the
very first day of class . . . and like it."
—Dr. Henry H. Heard

Studying for the Long Term: Developing a Deep Knowledge of Medicine

What's the best way to learn? This has been studied in
chess players, musicians, ER physicians, and athletes.
Is it where you are educated? Is it your experience? Is it
domain-specific training?

All of these are factors, yet none of them really
determine mastery. The people who learn the most and
who learn the quickest are those who employ what is
called *deliberate practice*. Deliberate practice is also
known as metacognition. It's thinking about your own
thinking. Someone who uses deliberate practice thinks
constantly about where they're weak, where they want to
go, and what they have to learn to get there.

Throughout your PA school experience, you will want
to use deliberate practice and think very hard about your
own thinking and learning. In this chapter, let's explore
how you can do that.

Here's the holy grail of medical knowledge: the four questions that drive understanding. There are four questions that will drive your understanding of medicine, and this is very, very important. This is your home base. This is where it's all got to come back to when it comes to learning any disease process. Throughout PA school, you're going to learn anatomy, physiology, epidemiology, and general sciences. But when it comes right down to it, your ultimate aim is to then take what you learn and apply it to disease states. With every single disease state, your thinking has always got to come back to four questions.

The first question is *pathophysiology*. What physiological processes are associated with a given disease? What is going wrong in the body? If a patient has strep throat, you need to understand what is actually wrong with the body. You need to be able to close your book and know automatically that strep throat comes from beta-hemolytic strep, known as *streptococcus pyogenes*. This bacterium affects the throat because the throat has receptors in it that render it very prone to this pharyngitis.

The second question is presentation. How is the patient going to present—what are the symptoms? If the patient has strep throat, she will come in complaining of fever, headache, and a sore throat.

The third question asks about diagnosis. How do you diagnose strep throat? Is it from a physical exam? Is it by history? Is it by diagnostic tests, like a rapid strep test, a throat culture, or a blood test? You need to know how to make a definitive diagnosis, whether that entails a clinical diagnosis, a diagnostic test, or a menagerie of tests to be aligned in order to establish a diagnosis.

Fourth and finally, you need to ask and answer the

question of treatment. How do you treat a given disease state? With an antibiotic? By admitting the patient to the hospital? With counseling?

With every single disease state, you must work your way through these four questions.

Strive for long-term, holistic understanding and knowledge. Adult learners have to hear things and study things approximately six times before they memorize them for the long term. What does that mean? It means that you can't learn about or study congestive heart failure one time and think you have mastery over that disease process.

When people try to study everything at once, it causes system overload. This is called informational blindness. You get so much information that the brain can't take it all in, so instead the brain just shuts off. This isn't just counterproductive, it's also demoralizing. A complicated topic is a pyramid. You need to learn a base amount of information and constantly stack on top of it. When you learn a song, you always learn the refrain first, and then you start filling in the verses. You need to learn the basic fundamentals of the disease process and then constantly keep fine-tuning that knowledge. There's a ton of knowledge you need to absorb, and you need to take that knowledge in manageable serving sizes.

So how do you know what the base of the pyramid is? It goes back to the four questions: what are the disease state's pathophysiology, presentation, diagnosis, and treatment? You need to understand the very common presentation of the disease, the common pathology of the disease, common ways to diagnose the disease, and common ways to treat the disease, and only after you have all this information down pat should you begin worrying about less common presentations, treatments, and so on. Guys, you've got to come back to congestive heart failure not once, not twice, but twenty times, always adding a little more to your base of information.

Throughout PA school and on your rotations, you have to consistently be making investments into your knowledge. If you do not do this, then when it comes time to take your boards, you will be at a significant disadvantage.

> *"Get a PANCE review book early that is broken down into categories. You can go through each section while you're learning it in the didactic classes. Professors give you so much information during didactic classes, but using a review book will help you really know what to focus on."*
> —Maddie Windstein

When you don't understand something, stop the line.
If a car is being built and going through an assembly line and something is wrong on the car, you need to stop the assembly line. You pull the cord and the conveyor belt stops, and you fix the problem. For a long time this was encouraged practice in Japanese auto manufacturing, where anyone who stopped the line was rewarded, whereas in American car manufacturing, workers never stopped the line for anything, because stopping the line cost something insane like $40,000 per minute. This had a major impact on the automotive industry.

I think that same phenomenon, a fear of stopping the line, often happens when PA students are studying. They don't stop the line when something is wrong. People will hear a term and not know what it means, but they don't stop the line to say, "Wait a second, let me try to figure out exactly what this means." They just kind of go, "I get the gist of it." You may think you get the gist of it, but you need to know more than just the gist; you need to know *everything*. If you're studying and don't absolutely, completely understand a term, then you stop and look it up. If you're in lecture, you raise your hand and you say, "I don't understand that term."

Too many people leave little blind spots in their knowledge, and they don't quite understand the disease process because of those blind spots. One word or phrase can definitely impact a situation. If someone is in a hyper-sympathetic state, it means he has too much adrenaline running through his body, and if someone has too much adrenaline running through his body, he is going to have a fast heart rate, tachycardia, and hypertension. Well, if I said to you, "Any patient who is in alcohol withdrawal will be in a hyper-sympathetic state," and if you don't understand that term "hyper-sympathetic state," then you won't know that a heart rate of 120 and blood pressure of 190/110 represents a hyper-sympathetic state, you may miss a question about alcohol withdrawal on a test, and more importantly, you may not be able to diagnose patients in the future.

Be very stubborn about correcting your blind spots. You are not going to hear something you don't understand and be passive about it. You are going to be proactive to fix the holes in your knowledge.

Set specific, measurable goals. People who employ deliberate practice set goals. They always are asking,

"What do I most want to learn from this course? How will I improve my knowledge retention? What do I want out of this rotation? What are three things that I hope to gain from this rotation?" They're constantly looking at their life, determining what do they want to do, and assessing their progress.

I cannot stress enough how important goals are. If I was a PA school program director, I would make goal setting mandatory. I want you to set goals and put them in writing. These goals could be physical, emotional, spiritual, or intellectual.

These goals set your mind on a course of what's called *synchrodestiny*: once you plan out your future, life will conspire with you to realize your goals. I'm not quoting a textbook or spouting psychological babble. I'm saying this has been the experience of my life.

Say you decide you're going to buy a Jeep Grand Cherokee. You say to yourself, "You know? Yep. That's the kind of car I want to buy when I graduate." Then what happens is, every time a Jeep drives by, you're going to look at it. It's going to stick in your subconscious and serve as fuel for the fire when it comes to your goal. You're going to decide not to buy coffee that day and put another five bucks in your car fund, and you're going to get to your goal much more quickly than you would have had you not put it into words and put it on paper.

I recommend one-year goals, three-year goals, five-year goals, ten-year goals, and twenty-year goals. When you go on rotations, you may even have weekly goals. Members of the graduating class of Yale in the 1970s were asked a series of questions. One of the questions was, "Who in here has a written set of goals?" Only 3 percent of the students did. This study was followed up on twenty years later, and the 3 percent of students who'd had written goals were found to have a higher quality of life, a subjective measure, and to be making more money than their peers, an objective measure.

Goals are magical, and they're the basis of deliberate practice.

Gain and maintain self-awareness. In addition to being reflective, be tough on yourself. A key leadership trait is self-awareness. You need to know who you are. You need to know where you come from. You need to look in the nooks and crannies of yourself and realize where you fall short, where you're driven by pride or ego.

A delusion is when something is true, but you cannot see or believe it is true. Also, the more the truth is pointed out to you, the harder and more aggressively you work to avoid seeing it.

For example, I liked to believe I was still one hundred and ninety pounds with six-pack abs, capable of doing ultra-endurance events and kickboxing like I did when I was in my thirties. I really identified that way. The truth, however, became painfully obvious when I started an exercise program. The first step of the exercise program was to take a picture of myself with my shirt off. The picture clearly showed a middle-aged guy who had gotten out of shape. This picture pissed me off and disturbed me to an unbelievable degree, because it highlighted my delusion and forced me to look at the truth.

So what did I do? I made the picture the screensaver on my phone. I forced myself to look at my delusion, and this strategy was very effective at getting me to work out and return to eating in more healthful way.

Without true awareness, your growth is going to be extremely limited, and to a huge degree you're going to be living a facade. This kind of awareness may require meditation, prayer, and outside input. Perhaps you think you're an extremely objective person with no delusions. The people who say this are typically the most subjective. You have to identify the garbage and biases in your head; this will help you become more self-aware and able to transform yourself. This kind of self-awareness lies at the heart of leadership and deliberate practice.

A student might think that because she's been a straight-A student her whole life, PA school should come easily for her. Another student might think that because he worked on an ambulance, he knows his stuff better than anybody else. Somebody may be coming into PA school as a nurse and thinking that puts her ahead of everybody else. All sorts of people have biases that may impact their patient interactions.

When people come to PA school with the delusion of self-importance or arrogance, their ability to serve their patients is diminished. Learning medicine is all about humility. Yes, you need confidence, but you also need humility. When it comes to delusions, you must be very honest about your own blind spots—you must develop a keen self-awareness. You are learning medicine, and you need to stay humble and hungry.

Develop unconscious competence. When it comes to studying for life, there are four different quadrants. They are unconscious incompetence, conscious incompetence, conscious competence, then unconscious competence. Let me explain.

Unconscious incompetence means you're not even aware you don't know or can't do something. For instance, a baby doesn't know that it can't walk. The second phase is conscious incompetence. This means at least you know where you're weak. You know where you're ignorant, and then you can go to work. A baby, once he decides to try walking, tries to stand up long before his legs are strong enough. So you work at it, and then you go to the next phase, which is conscious competence: you know it if you can deeply think about it; you have to really focus. Once a baby learns to walk, he has to really work at it, balancing and wobbling. The last phase is unconscious competence, where you know it like the back of your hand. Eventually, walking becomes second nature.

In medicine, developing unconscious competence—competence to the degree that you can do your job without having to think about it—involves way more than just time and energy. Your learning has got to be *smart* learning. There's no question that repetition is a factor, and repetition of high-quality information will give you that unconscious competence, but in order to develop this kind of competence, you need that good old metacognition: deliberate practice, thinking about your own thinking.

Think about what you need to know, what you need to learn, and where you are weak. Set goals and reevaluate your performance. You must always ask yourself, "What about this topic needs to be second nature to me? What do I need to know like the back of my hand?"

Say you identify a need to have unconscious competence when it comes to knowing the causes of chest pain. From there, you develop a system in which you are constantly reviewing these causes of chest pain whenever you see a patient with chest pain. When you miss certain causes, you need to be quick to identify your errors, and you need to be vigilant in correcting those errors in the future.

Be tough on yourself. Say you see a patient and afterwards, you ask yourself, "How did I do there?" You did okay, John, but you didn't give the patient aspirin. "Oh crap, that's right, I didn't give them aspirin." The next time you're in that situation, you sure won't forget the aspirin. Make sure you have a cognitive checklist of the things that you're supposed to do; as you do this time and time again, thinking about where you dropped the ball, after a while you realize you are doing everything exactly and perfectly as you should. You are unconsciously competent.

The methods that work best for you when it comes to developing that unconscious competence will in part dictate your study tactics. I found I had to use flashcards. So I would take a body of information, convert it to flashcards, and then flip through the flashcards. Some people may say, "Well, John, that is very inefficient, that is very slow," and from a time perspective I guess it was—but I would master the information. This method allowed me to develop unconscious competence. So it might have been slow, but it was very effective. Always be asking yourself not only what material you need to know, but also how you specifically need to learn it. Do you have to open up the book? Do you have to again convert to flashcards? Do you have to watch YouTube videos? Figuring out what works best for you is part of the metacognitive aspect of developing unconscious competence.

Study Smarter

Understand and value the syllabus. For each class, your syllabus will tell you the course objectives, what your instructor will cover in the course, when office hours are, and how your grade will actually be assessed. If you're like me before PA school, and even during PA school, you may think the syllabus is a pain in the butt. You get the syllabus and you file it away. You want to know when tests are going to be, but you don't really go through the syllabus in detail or refer back to it.

What I'm about to mention makes people very uncomfortable to talk about, but you should know. It is not uncommon for PA students who get decelerated or kicked out of PA school to lawyer up and try to get back into PA school. Should that happen, the syllabus serves as a contract, and a student's case can depend on whether or not the teacher and/or the student followed or deviated from that contract. You must understand that the syllabus is a contract between you and the college. It's a really big deal.

Hopefully you will never find yourself in that situation—but even so, you must study and understand each syllabus very well. At minimum, you will then have a thorough understanding of how the instructors plan to grade and assess you.

Find your study group. There are some studies behind how long people can stay in a cold body of water—if other people are with you, you last longer than if you're struggling by yourself. There is strength in unity. I do not recommend being a lone wolf in PA school. Join a pack. It allows the studying to be more efficient and more effective. Study groups are also important for your emotional welfare, because the studying can be brutal. I formed my closest relationships in PA school in my study group. We would study together all the time. We'd study early in the morning; we'd have lunch together; we'd study after hours together. We were able to compare notes, share our strengths, and pool our resources. I absolutely loved it. We became very close, and we were there for each other. This allowed us to watch out for each other and help each other when one of us struggled—everyone goes through low points in PA school.

You've got to really like the people in your study group, and you've got to have synergistic core values. Some groups are more fun and social, and others are very academic, made of take-no-prisoners bookworms. I think it is really important to find a group that studies with your same values, and finding that group may take some amount of trial and error. Don't be afraid to leave a study group that is not serving your needs.

When you get together, you need to have set rules and systems for how you will study. I cannot stress this enough. You need to be prioritizing those four questions of medicine: pathophysiology, presentation, diagnosis, and treatment. In my study group, we would take our notes from the day and we would read our notes to each other, going around in a circle. One person would read her section, and we would all follow along in our own notes. Any time we had questions about something or conflicting information, we would stop and look up a topic and make sure we all understood.

I recommend scheduling breaks for your study group— whether short ten-minute walks that will help you clear your heads, or longer and more social breaks that will help you sharpen the saw. In my study group, we would alternate who made Sunday dinner for the rest of the group, and then we would study afterwards. Study groups are great to plan social events or exercise events with outside of study time.

Understand and capitalize on your learning style.
Different people learn in different ways. Some people are verbal learners, meaning that they do well with written and spoken words. Visual learners, on the other hand, gravitate towards images and spatial information. Aural/audio learners prefer to learn by hearing information, whether through spoken language or music. Kinesthetic/physical learners are those who learn best using their sense of touch and movement. Finally, some people learn better in solitary environments, whereas others learn optimally in social environments where they're able to discuss concepts with others.

Traditional study styles—opening a book and reviewing notes—typically work well for verbal learners. For visual learners, one good option is to go to YouTube, because someone has probably made some kind of video that explains the topic at hand in a way that will provide an aha moment. (I should mention here that I have more than five hundred videos on YouTube explaining all sorts of concepts and providing tools for learning medicine.) Of course, you will want to ensure that the source you find is credible. If you are a visual learner working on learning a topic and you just can't quite get it, you may benefit from taking out a poster board and drawing or mind-mapping the relevant parts of the topic.

If you are having problems memorizing key concepts, that is when flashcards are very important, especially for visual and kinesthetic learners. I think it is really important that you create and use flashcards in a very specific way. A flashcard is not an opportunity to rewrite your notes. That is not what flashcards are for. Flashcards are for key concepts with very specific names; you can have a bulky question on one side, but all you want on the back is a very clean answer. I also recommend using different colors. I would always write the question in pen and the answer in marker. This changed both how I wrote and how I read the question and answer. This strategy engaged my visual sense, and moving the cards around also engaged my kinesthetic sense. Some people may say that writing out flashcards is terribly inefficient. Again, what is actually inefficient is when you don't know your stuff.

For audio learners, be sure you have and use a good digital recorder. If instructors allow you to record the class, you can listen to the recording whenever it is convenient for you, take notes at different points, and even record your notes and listen to those.

Kinesthetic learners can also be helped by using their bodies to learn concepts. I could use my left hand, make a fist, extend my pinkie, and form a gun with my pointer finger and my thumb in order to describe and picture my coronary blood vessels. Or, to remember the twelve causes of secondary hypertension, I could go head to toe pointing out all the potential causes in a very sequential pattern, until gradually this knowledge became automatic. Some kinesthetic learners even benefit a great deal from tossing a ball against the wall or squeezing a relaxation ball as they study.

"Students who are successful in the didactic phase understand what their personal learning style is and how to manage their time effectively. Due to the arduous pace, staying ahead of your studies is important—playing catch-up is near impossible."
—Kristin Thomson

Utilize all your available time. NET time is No Extra Time. What does that mean? It means if you drive forty-five minutes to school and forty-five minutes home, guess what? You've got an hour and a half each day to study, if you so choose to do so, by listening to audio notes or lecture recordings. Utilize all of the time you possibly can.

It should be mentioned that multitasking has been proven not to work very well when it comes to combining two or more tasks that require considerable cognitive attention. This means that the trick with NET is to incorporate a task that does require cognitive attention—studying—into a task that does *not* require cognitive attention. Any time you are doing something relatively automatic that you would be doing anyway—working out on the elliptical, driving, or walking to the store—you can be utilizing NET.

Take active notes. There are some very good studies out of UCLA and Stanford that say if you take very good notes, your recall goes up 50 percent. I've seen this in my live conferences, and I've seen it personally.

If you really want to learn thoroughly, take very good notes, and then convert your notes to another notebook, interpreting and commenting on your initial notes. Folks, that's an absolute key feature of a disciplined study plan. Too many people go to a PowerPoint presentation, and they read the PowerPoint and call it a day—but that's very passive learning. You don't retain information in the long term using that kind of strategy, and the literature reflects that. Take notes on your notes. Write down connections you observe, highlight anything you don't understand that you need to follow up on, and continue practicing that good old metacognition about the material and your learning process.

Don't allow yourself to get distracted. For the duration of PA school, from your didactic phase to when you take your boards, you'll need a disciplined study plan. As a business owner and entrepreneur, I study business literature often. I remember reading somewhere that one hour of uninterrupted study time equals 2.6 hours of interrupted time.

That's why, in generating this book for you, I'm at the office alone on a Saturday morning. I can get more work done in one hour, sitting in the office by myself, than I could at home, where I would be answering phone calls, seeing emails, getting interrupted by my wife and kids, and feeling like I should take out the garbage or walk my dog.

You need to get away from your spouse, your kids, your roommate, or whoever you live with. You need to turn off your phone so you don't take texts. If you listen to music, make sure it does not have lyrics in it, because if you're hearing lyrics in a song, especially a song that you really like, your focus is going to be divided.

Studying is like doing chest compressions in CPR. You need to do about twenty chest compressions before you build up enough perfusion pressure that each compression squirts out blood to perfuse the heart. As soon as you come off of the chest, perfusion pressure drops as fast as mercury drops when you open a bezel on a blood pressure cuff. When you're studying, you're getting it, you're getting it, you're getting it, you're growing—and then you get a text, you get completely distracted, and it takes you ten minutes to get back into the groove.

Get alone, find some quiet space, focus your studying, and optimize your retention.

Test Taking 101

By now you know that you cannot and will not be a victim of your grades; you know that you are in control of your learning and your destiny. Here's the key, though, ladies and gentlemen. If you asked me, "John, how do I get really good grades in PA school?" I would not respond, "Learn the medicine really well." That's only about 60 percent of it. You have to learn how to play the game.

Know your instructor. You need to understand how your teachers test. You have to understand where the test comes from and how the questions are made. The same will be true when you are preparing for your boards. Where are your teachers getting their test questions, and how are they testing you? If they're using tests from past classes, it would be unethical for you to ask senior classmates for specific details about the tests, but you can inquire about trends. Do teachers pull from test banks? Do they use open-ended questions?

You need to study the techniques that your instructor employs to test you, and you need to play the game well. Remember that PA school is a social system, with patterns associated with memorization and manipulation of information. Of course you want to develop a deep knowledge of medicine that stands up to real-world practice—but that won't mean a hill of beans if you can't play the game and get passing grades. I need you to study your faculty members, study their testing techniques, and play ball well.

Look for patterns. I remember the one test I failed in PA school—it was a psychiatry final exam. I had the opportunity to retake the test, and when I went back and started studying the material, I looked at all of the tests from this particular professor. I realized, looking at all of his multiple-choice pretests, that he never designated choice A as an answer, not one single time. He had, clearly, a bias against A. I also noticed that he loved the letter C. I have since learned that C as the correct answer is a trend among test creators. This particular professor chose the letter C as the correct response approximately 60 percent of time. When I took the test again, I was able to eliminate A, and when I didn't know the correct answer, I would pick C.

I ended up getting 100 percent on the retest, not because I knew all the information—although I certainly knew more than I had the first time—but because I had studied the tester. I'm going to say this again: PA school is a social system, and you have to learn to play the game.

Common Issues During the Didactic Phase

*"By the time a student has been accepted to a PA
program they have proven that they are capable of
completing the program. But they must keep their eye
on the ball from the first day of class to the end of
the program. There are a few things that sometimes
happen to students, their close friends, or their family
that can cause them to take their eye off of the ball
and stumble. This often presents as a drop in their
academic performance. These things include Death,
Disease, Divorce (or relationship problems), Drugs
(or alcohol), Dollars, Diapers, Deployment, Distance,
Dependents, and Dysfunctional coping skills. So it
pays to have a good support network."*
—Dr. Robert Philpot

Deal with life events that crop up. Things happen in
life, and many things can happen during your time in PA
school that add to your already considerable stress and
threaten to throw you off course. Divorces, pregnancies,
and deaths happen during PA school, like they do at any
other time. Now is not the time to grin and bear it. Now is
the time to have a closed-door meeting with your advisor
or the program director. My advice is to disclose your
situation early and have the program assess where you
stand. If all of a sudden your spouse moves out and you
start decompensating, and you get worse for a month and
eventually your grades are in the crapper, you may have
a very difficult time salvaging your year. Go immediately to
the program and let them know what is going on.

Get help for any learning and testing challenges you may have. Resources for those with learning difficulties will vary from school to school. If you know or suspect you have a learning disability, you will want to go through the necessary channels to assess and document that disability so that you are able to receive accommodations such as more testing time or private testing. If you don't go through the proper administrative channels, you will have a tough time getting sympathy from a faculty member, and you may not have much recourse if your grades turn sour.

> *"If you are struggling, get help—your advisors, tutors, academic resource centers, and cognitive skills centers. Make maximum use of every resource available to you."*
> —Christopher Hanifin

Manage your anxiety. Anxiety in the didactic phase is a rite of passage. Studying and test taking are difficult and stressful, yes, but try to remember again that this is not about you—it is about your future patients. Being a PA can be a stressful profession, and you are going to be in situations—having demanding docs coming down on you, being in the position to affect a patient's well-being—that are a thousand times more stressful than a test.

I don't mean to sound unfeeling, but if you are unable to manage the kind of anxiety that you experience during the didactic year, you are in for even worse down the line. Whatever anxiety you have during your didactic year will pale in comparison to what you'll experience preparing for your board exams, so my advice is that you begin practicing anxiety management now. Try to keep things in perspective, take care of your mind and body, seek out the support of your loved ones, and keep on keeping on. If you need to see a counselor and get appropriate treatment, you should certainly do so.

Address burnout head-on. In the didactic year, burnout is a very real phenomenon as you study and work constantly. Pretty much every semester, both in college and PA school, I studied incredibly aggressively and then at some point experienced what I called my "drought." I would have a week or two where I just couldn't study anymore. For me this happened about 60 percent of the way through the semester. I would want to study, and I would need to study, but I couldn't. I had no drive. The only thing that worked was to surrender and stop studying. I found that the quickest way for me to get out of my drought was basically to say, "Well, I hope I don't do much damage until this drought is over." I went fishing; I exercised. In my experience, this made the drought go away more quickly.

Some Final Words of Wisdom for Your Didactic Year . . .

"Some of my more favorite dictums in the didactic phase include:
- *Re: the physical exam: 'Make it flow from head to toe.'*
- *How I do depends upon what I did.*
- *After thirty-five years of ER experience: 'A needle, in health care, is just like a saw; it will rear up and bite you if you turn your back on it.'*

■ *Ticks are like ninjas: You often don't see them because they hide in the shadows."*

—Dr. Gary B. Tooley

"Organize your priorities in a way to meet the many demands of life, and be sure to schedule time with family and friends."

—Wallace Boeve

"Recognize that the faculty are utterly on your side— they want you to succeed. Sometimes it is easy for an 'us vs. them' mentality to develop between the students and the faculty. The faculty are on your team. It is their job to challenge you and push you outside of your comfort zones. When you think a faculty member is riding you hard, consider this: If you hired a personal fitness trainer and they did not push you hard, what would you do? You would fire them. Accept that you are investing tremendous time, money, and effort into your education, and be thankful for the faculty that push you. They see something in you."

—Christopher Hanifin

"To survive and thrive in the didactic year, create a study plan for each class and build in some time to relax/exercise/go to the movies or whatever you do to de-stress. Limit the use of alcohol as a de-stressor. If your study plan and technique is not working well, seek out your advisor or a course director and ask for assistance! Your faculty is there to assist you! Don't expect perfection or straight A's. Do your best

and accept there is always more to learn!"
—Nancy Hurwitz

"You need to have two Fs in PA education: Flexibility: You will be working in medicine, so get used to changing schedules, missed appointments, and working late into the evening or weekend. Clinical faculty might be late for a class due to problems with their patients, clinics, or ORs running late. Focus: Become task-oriented. Complete assignments in a timely fashion, and never fall behind. Check for errors in all of your work. Some social activities may have to go on the backburner for the next two years."
—Richard E. Murphy

"Success means time management, not memorizing material but understanding it, and developing excellent interpersonal communications skills."
—Dr. James Kilgore

Chapter 3

Your Second Year: The Clinical Phase

"Be willing to arrive early, stay late, and participate in everything—an overall 'willingness attitude' will open many opportunities down the road."
—Wallace Boeve

During rotations, you will be spending three- to four-week intervals at clinical facilities in various areas of medicine: pediatrics, surgery, gynecology, and others. Rotations are an extremely exciting time where you actually get to apply what you've learned. It's a wonderful time to learn how to engage with physicians, nurses, and patients and practice the art of medicine in a controlled setting. This is the right time to make mistakes.

Your rotations give you an opportunity to learn medicine like you'll never have again in your life once you have graduated. On my surgical rotation, I made it a point to learn as much as I possibly could. I came in an hour early and started all the IVs for the nursing staff; they loved me, and I gained valuable practice. I would work a ten- or twelve-hour surgical shift in the OR, and when I finished, I would ask the ER doc if I could come down to the ER for a couple of hours. It was just free learning.

As a PA, you're like a teenager driving your car on your parents' insurance. That kind of protection goes away when you graduate, so you should take advantage of it—do not be a passive learner. Be a proactive learner.

Rotations will also help you gain insight into which area you feel pulled to, which is always very individual. You may discover that you are passionate about an area you hadn't really considered. It is not uncommon for someone to say, "You know, I thought I never wanted to go deal with kids, but I was inspired by my pediatrics preceptor and had an amazing pediatrics rotation." I encourage you to keep an open mind during rotations, rather than going into them with a preconceived notion of where you are headed.

Mindset, Revisited

As you prepare to begin your rotations, I want you to revisit your mindset. It will be very important for you to be focused, positive, proactive, and open-minded as you continue to learn and as you interact with a wide range of people.

Revisit your goals and mission statement. I highly recommend that you have a written set of goals and objectives—as always, for life in general, but also for your goals that are specific to rotations. On rotations, clearly, you're focused on your intellectual goals, things that you want to learn. "I want to learn EKGs on a scale of 9 out of 10. I want to learn all the arrhythmias that are going to be on my boards. I want to learn how to assess someone with chest pain. I want to learn the twenty most common antibiotics prescribed in family practice or primary care." Also, revisit your mission statement. How has it evolved? How can you align your goals with your mission statement?

Always be learning. When you first go on rotations, you will learn how to suture, and the first time you suture, it's going to be incredibly exciting. You are going from the academic classroom, where you probably learned on pigs' feet, to a clinical environment where you are putting sutures in a human being. You open up your suture kit, you put on your sterile gloves, and you feel like you're a doctor on TV. But after you start suturing five times, ten times, twenty times, thirty times, your learning curve, which has been climbing, begins to level out. Your curve begins to become a horizontal line.

Your brain is no longer open to taking in new information, and that's when you're done; that's when you've closed the door to new information, and that's where you stop developing as a clinician.

Always keep your brain about 10 percent open to new learning, and that's in all areas of your life. Who knows what else there is to know about suturing? How can you continue to develop your technique to take into account different body types and body parts? Continue to be observant; continue to ask questions and do research.

Do not fall into the trap of being closed-minded. Continue practicing metacognition and self-awareness.

Don't be afraid to look stupid. The biggest mistake PA students make going on rotations is a mistake that has been perpetuated throughout the academic system on a wide scale. People are afraid to look stupid. People are afraid to make mistakes and afraid to be wrong, and this extremely limits their growth.

I hope you can hear what I'm saying. I meet a lot of college students who are so afraid of being wrong that they won't speak up in class, or they won't fully engage during their rotations. They are people who are going to be extremely limited in their careers, because medicine is all about growth. It's all about learning through trial and error. Remember, if you make a mistake, there's always going to be someone there to help you.

Be decisive and aim for completion. My advice is, "Go for it." Do not be afraid to be wrong. This is the exact right time to be wrong.

When you are on rotations, you will be writing SOAP reports—Subjective, Objective, Assessment, and Plan—in which you get the patient's subjective input, gather objective data, make a diagnosis, and determine next steps. What I've found after precepting approximately fifty students is that students get really good at presenting me with half of a SOAP report. Students are confident in information gathering and testing, but they hesitate to be wrong when it comes to interpreting the information.

A lot of times, PA students do better at more by-the-book physical exams than I do, as they are being meticulous and have studied all of this in depth. But when it comes to the assessment and plan, students often come to me without an idea of where to go. "I don't know what to do with this one," students say to me all the time.

My advice is this: For 100 percent of the patients you see, I want an assessment and plan. What does this mean? It means that you're always thinking things through and making up your mind. I would rather have a student think everything through and be drastically wrong than come to me without an understanding of where to go, without wanting to put themselves out there.

go for it!

54

That kind of trepidation will delay your growth significantly. Students who are willing to say, "This is what I want to do. If I were a PA, this is what I would do today"—they are very easy to fix. They have the right strategy, the right mindset, and the right critical thinking skills, and over the course of their rotations, they will be right more and more of the time as they learn from their errors.

The problem comes when you go through PA school passive, with blinders on, too afraid to make up your mind. In that case, you will get out of PA school and spend the next three years trying to catch up, trying to gain those critical thinking skills required to make decisions and the confidence required to implement plans.

This is really important. Always, always make sure your mindset is one of completion. Do not be afraid to be wrong. Again, your clinical year is like driving on your parents' permit. Your insurance is covered, so if you crash your car, it's not going on your permanent record.

How to Succeed in Rotations

Understand that as soon as you get on rotation, there will be questions asked of you within the first five minutes. You're going to put your stuff down, put your stethoscope around your neck, and get your first patient. Some students, particularly very introverted students, might have a tough time transitioning to rotations. If you like flying under the radar, or if you have any personality difficulties, you are going to need to adjust to the highly personal nature of rotations.

Continue your study habits in preparation for the boards. Understand that you still have to study, guys. When you're on rotations, you have to study, you have to study, you have to study. The rotations are not a time for partying.

I remember once—when I was working on an ambulance before starting PA school—I was talking to a PA student who was on rotations. This PA student said, "Oh, this is great. I've been on rotations. I haven't cracked a book for months." That's the kiss of death when it comes to your boards and when it comes to developing real knowledge.

You need to study material for your rotations, and you also need to study for your boards beginning on day one of your rotations. Too many people get on rotations and crack the book just enough to keep in the good graces of the preceptor, or just enough to pass their end-of-rotation exams, but they neglect to study for their boards throughout their rotations.

If you don't study for your boards, your chances of failure are extremely high. When I teach board review courses, I ask people to be very honest about where they stand. I'll ask them, "Who partied on the rotations? Who cakewalked it? Who took it real easy?" I always see a lot of uncomfortable faces.

> *"Get a PANCE review book with plenty of practice questions. During down time, work on those questions that relate to the rotation you are on. That way if you don't understand, you have your supervising doctor to ask!"*
> —Maddie Windstein

Continue being a consummate professional. You have to understand that when you go on rotations, you're not just going there to learn medicine—you're also there to learn the political culture of working in the healthcare field. You'll be engaging with doctors, nurses, patients, and ancillary staff. This is going to be a tremendous learning process. First and foremost, when you are well-liked by your preceptor, every part of your job goes better. From a business perspective, it is said that what interests my preceptor fascinates me.

I really encourage you to engage with your preceptor at a high level—and in a professional manner. You're not obligated to go out for drinks with your preceptor; you're not obligated to go hang out with your preceptor outside of the rotation.

I have seen some preceptors take advantage of students, using them to inflate their own ego or self-esteem. That is not your job. You're not there to make their job easier, and you're not there to validate them. You're there to learn.

Show up on time and prepared. Clearly, you can never be late for rotations. If you're not sure where your site is, do a drive-by and make sure you will be able to arrive, park, and get in at least ten to fifteen minutes early. If you are meeting with a surgeon at six a.m., for the love of Pete, get to the hospital at 5:15, grab a cup of coffee, and do some studying in the meantime.

Almost always before rotations, students are required to reach out to the preceptor to ask what time to show up and where to go. My advice would be for you also to ask the preceptor, "What is one thing I should study or know about before I show up on my first day?" (Don't ask, "Is there anything in particular I should study or know?" Be sure to word it so that the preceptor will be more likely to offer something: "*What is one thing* I should study or know?") That is an excellent way to get into the good graces of the preceptor. Then you have to bust your ass and make sure you really know whatever the preceptor mentions.

I would recommend that you have business cards made when you go on rotation—just simple cards with basic contact information and maybe a LinkedIn address—and give those out like candy. Also, constantly talk to physicians about job possibilities.

> "*Before you start each rotation, Google your rotation site and preceptor. Get to know as much as you can about them before you arrive. Also, review your study notes on that area of medicine. Don't go into a surgery rotation not knowing your anatomy or surgical instruments. It makes you and the program look bad.*"
> —Deborah Summers

Cultivate enthusiasm, respect, and a commitment to learning. I cannot make this clearer: I love students who *really want to learn*. How do I know if a student wants to learn? I notice when students display proactivity, positivity, and the other elements we've covered. But I love a student who's got a notepad.

If I bring up something—"Hey, the EKG findings of hyperkalemia are peaked T waves"—and a student pulls out a notebook and writes it down, I think that's wonderful. I think, "Oh, I've got a good student here. I've got someone who really wants to learn."

Whatever you do, do not say, "Oh, I already knew that." That makes the preceptor think they're wasting your time, wasting your precious and knowledgeable time, because you already knew something. The last thing you want to do is shut your preceptor down from teaching.

Yes, you may be textbook smart, but you don't have the experience that your preceptor does. You haven't lived in the trenches and crossed through the battlegrounds. Don't ever say to a preceptor, "Oh, I already knew that."

If they ask you specifically whether you know something, of course you should be honest, but you can still display humility and a desire to learn. You can say, "I know that from a textbook, but I still really want the clinical knowledge. That's more important to me." Or you can say, "I know some aspects of that topic, but I would be eager to fill in the gaps." You want to keep encouraging your preceptors to teach you.

One of the first questions your preceptors will ask is, "What do you think you want to do when you graduate?" Here, your preceptor is trying to gauge your interest in the current rotation and area of medicine. If you're doing a pediatrics rotation, the preceptor wants to know if there's a chance you're going to end up in pediatrics. How much time and energy should they invest in your knowledge? Whatever you do, do not say, "Oh, I want to do anything but this." If you said that to me, or indicated in any way that you were unenthused about your rotation with me, I would sit you in the corner for four weeks.

You've got to keep an open mind, not only because you never know what you'll end up liking, but also because you want to keep your preceptor engaged with your learning. If you go onto a urology rotation, the urologist wants to see whether you would be a good cultural fit. Should they train you so well that if they wanted to hire you, their investment would pay off? So when the urologist says, "Well, what do you think you want to do when you graduate?" you say, "Urology seems like an extraordinary profession. It's been on my mind. I think rectal exams twenty times a day might be a good thing for me. It seems like the quality of life would be extraordinary, so I've really considered urology."

Do I encourage being deceptive? No, I don't—yet I want you to be smart, politically savvy, and open-minded. Keep your future full of possibilities. Say, "I've really considered urology. I'm really looking forward to this rotation."

> *"It might not seem like it while you are in school, but PA school is very short and goes by amazingly quickly. Make good use of your time, and see as many patients as possible. As a student on an inpatient service, you will often only be assigned a couple of patients to follow each day. Know every single patient on the floor, whether they are 'yours' or not. If someone comes in with a murmur or a big liver, make sure you get in the room with them. Arrive early and stay late. You only have one shot at PA school. Be aggressive."*
> —Christopher Hanifin

Know and use the proper etiquette. Please remember that you are a guest. You are a guest in a facility. Everybody knows when there's a PA student in the house. You're there with your short white coat on, and everyone knows you're a guest. You have that new car smell to you.

As a guest, you don't take any seat that's available; you ask where you should sit. You ask where you should put your jacket, and you ask where you should put your meals. You are always unfailingly polite. What I find with PA students is that they typically exhibit this politeness for the first couple of days, and then halfway through the rotation, they become very casual.

I'm saying stick with it—understand that you are not an asset, you are a liability and a distraction. This is not to say you can't contribute in positive ways. A very good student lights up any facility. When staff members know that you're respectful and driven and a pleasure to be around, it makes everything better.

If, on the other hand, you have a bad student—someone who's lazy, someone who's a little cantankerous, someone who is not polite—it sucks the life out of the facility and will really hurt your learning during your rotation. It's not uncommon for preceptors just to let a student like that sit in a corner and study for forty hours a week for their whole rotation if they're not well-liked.

Don't be a clock-watcher. Make sure you're always fifteen minutes early and stay as late as the learning continues. That's very important. I do not like clock-watchers; make sure you're there to learn and you're demonstrating your dedication to learning.

It is your job to go up and introduce yourself to every single person you see. If you don't know someone and haven't met them, you go introduce yourself and shake hands—whether it's the administrative assistant, the nurse, the nurse's aide, or the janitor. You shake that person's hand and say, "Hey, I'm a PA student from [whatever college you're from]. I'm going to be here for the next month. If you see anything interesting or cool that you think would be good for me to learn, please let me know. I would really appreciate it."

You will immediately get on the good side of everybody there, because they talk. That janitor may have been in that same hospital for thirty years, meaning he knows everybody, and once you've made a good impression, guess what? He is going to like you and say good things about you to other people.

You're going to have a lot of old-school docs who will not tolerate handheld devices. They have a negative connotation, and some docs will assume you are going to be lazy if you use them. Don't text, don't email, don't check your social media accounts, and if you're going to look at your phone, either go into the bathroom or ask permission, making clear that you're using it to support your learning. Say, "Hey, do you mind if I look something up really quick?" or, "I'd love to take some notes on what you just explained." As a general rule, do not look at your phone unless it's medically related, and even in that case, tell your preceptor what you're doing. And again, if you do need to send a personal email or text, go to the bathroom.

Request feedback and evaluation. Understand that a lot of preceptors do not like giving constructive criticism or telling you where you're falling short. This can be catastrophic for PAs, who can go through a rotation and think everything is going great. Then at the end of the rotation, they get lambasted on their evaluation and get a poor grade. A good preceptor, or a preceptor who has experience giving feedback, will give you feedback all along the way, so you'll have a very good idea of where you stand. But my experience is that this is not common, and most preceptors shy away from conflict.

The way you get around this is to ask for a mid-cycle evaluation. You go into your preceptor's office and say, "Listen, it's very important that I do a very good job during this rotation. I may not be able to see where I'm falling short of your expectations. I'd like to get a mid-cycle evaluation so you can tell me a couple of areas where I really need to improve before the end of this rotation."

Again, you have to assume that you're doing some things wrong or could stand to work on some areas. If you frame your question in a way that makes it easier to avoid giving criticism—"Are there major areas I need to work on?"—then it's likely your preceptor will indeed avoid giving criticism.

It's like if you're going to ask a patient if they're taking their medicines. You don't say, "Hey, are you taking your blood pressure pills as you should?" Because everybody is going to say, "Yes." You assume that they're not, and you ask the question like this: How often do you forget to take you blood pressure pills? Once a week? Twice a week?" You frame it in a way that allows them to give you a very honest answer.

When you go to your preceptor, you should say, "I know there are areas where I can improve. Where do you feel I need to improve most?" Guess what? Now you get a very open and honest answer.

Let's say your preceptor thinks you're horrible at your assessment and plan. Horrible. She may say, "Well, you may want to improve your assessment and plan." In that case, you go to work over the next two weeks in efforts to improve your assessment and plan.

Then let's say you show improvement, but you're still bad—not horrible, but pretty bad. Guess what? Your preceptor is still going to grade you based on the curve you've established. You're bad, but before you were horrible! As a result, your grade is still typically better than it would have been had you not solicited that feedback.

Choose your elective rotation carefully. During rotations, you'll have an elective rotation or even two, depending on your program, where you can pick whatever field you want to go into. This rotation is meant to help you explore your interests outside of the standard rotations. Nobody has to do a dermatology rotation, but let's say you grew up with bad acne and you want to get behind the curtain and see what goes on in dermatology—well, now you have the option to do your rotation in dermatology. I think the purpose of the elective rotation is really to expand the scope of your experience, to stretch yourself, and to see what is available.

If you're still considering your future focus and you want to take this elective to help you decide, that makes sense. But if you're already relatively sure what your focus will be, then my advice is to go a little crazy here. This is where you have an opportunity to go into a medical field that you really want to explore, even if that's not where you're going to end up. I could do an extra rotation, and I did mine in emergency medicine, so that I had two rotations in emergency medicine, my future focus. Looking back, I don't think I made the best choice; part of me wishes I had done something like cardiothoracic surgery where I could be more involved with heart surgery patients, or a rotation in pathology where I could help do autopsies on dead bodies and determine how they died. I wish I had done orthopedics, or dermatology, or ENT. This is the time to live out any dreams that may not be part of your future.

Exit each rotation gracefully and plan for the future.
At the end of each rotation, ask for a letter of reference, every single time. By the time you are done with your ten to twelve rotations, if you are away from the rotation site for four or five months, they forget about you. I precepted eight students per year, and even those I liked, respected, and remembered, I remembered far less well four or five months out than I did immediately after their rotations. So my advice is this: a week before the end of your rotation, ask for a favor and ask the preceptor to write you a letter of reference. The vast majority of preceptors will say yes, but some may dilly-dally or forget; you can ask again three days out and then one day out, and after that just let it go. By the time you are done with rotations, if you get a letter of reference from nine out of the twelve rotation sites, you can then pick three or four of the references that are your best to put into your resume. Only send the best ones.

It is not common to write thank-you notes to preceptors, but I think it should be mandatory. Thank your preceptor in a generic sense, and then thank them for one specific thing that made the biggest difference to you. This will make you more memorable to your preceptor.

Developing Patient Communication and Interaction

Remember that good medicine is *founded* on patient interaction. You have to understand that human nature and patient satisfaction determine good medicine. In other words, good medicine is determined by patient perception. If the patient thinks you did a good job, then guess what? You did a good job.

You have to understand that, in PA school and on rotations, you will be learning evidence-based medicine—a very left-brained, analytical approach. The problem is, patients do not care one bit about analytical, left-brained medicine. They assume you know your stuff, because you're a certified PA, or soon will be. What they care about is how you make them feel.

There's a big movement right now about patient satisfaction and hospital reimbursement, so this is currently a really hot topic among administrators, because even a medium-sized hospital can lose millions of dollars if patient satisfaction scores are low.

In addition to the concept that patient satisfaction means good medicine, it's very clear that angry patients are the ones who sue, whereas happy patients who like you don't sue. I have met with different attorneys, both plaintiff and defensive, and asked them both, "Why do medical malpractice claims happen?" It is interesting that both of them said the same thing. They said the biggest cause of these claims is poor communication. Patients don't feel like they got the case or complications explained to them well, they get angry, and that triggers a suit.

So engaging patients at a very high level is not only good for your career and your longevity, it's also good to decrease lawsuits—it's just plain good to have the patients like you. It's the greatest feeling when someone comes in and says, "Hey, you saw me six months ago, I'm so glad that you're on duty again." It's a great feeling when a patient likes you so much that they say, "Hey, do you have your own practice outside of the hospital?" That's when you know you've really exceeded expectations.

How do you exceed expectations? How do you engage patients in a way that your patient satisfaction scores go off the charts? First and foremost, you have to realize that it's important. You have to realize that when patients like you, every part of your job becomes easier.

> *"You cannot text a patient to figure out what is wrong with them. Developing the ability to communicate well with others and knowing the right questions to ask to determine their problem is a skill that every new PA must master to be a successful clinician."*
> —Dr. James Kilgore

Examine your biases. I want to share a quote from Herbert Spencer, a great thinker from the 1800s. He said, "There is a principle which is a bar against all information, which is proof against all argument, and which cannot fail to keep a man in everlasting ignorance. That principle is contempt prior to investigation." You will deal with many people, especially patients, about whom you have preconceived negative notions. Say a patient comes into the ER with fibromyalgia, back pain, and an allergy to ibuprofen and tramadol. It is very easy to look back at the patient's old records and see this person comes in constantly, and then to assume that the person is an addict just looking for an opiate. It is very easy to walk into the room with a real bias against that patient and some degree of contempt, even before you interact with the patient.

I'm going to stress, ladies and gentlemen, that you have to fight to keep an open mind. You have to fight, every time you walk into a patient's room, to clear your head, take a deep breath, and say to yourself, "I want to take this information that I know and assess it anew with a good history and a good physical exam." You have to fight the urge to make up your mind on a diagnosis or a treatment plan before you actually see the patient. Otherwise, you risk making misdiagnoses based on your assumptions, and you risk putting the patient at a distance from you and dissolving trust.

Build trust. How do you become well-liked by your patients? You have to keep in mind what I call the TLC score. You need to have an attitude of tender loving care towards your patients. You need to care for them even though they may not care for themselves.

- **Tone:** The T in TLC stands for tone. In the book *Blink*, by Malcolm Gladwell, Gladwell looks at two separate groups of surgeons. The surgeons in one group have been sued two or more times, and those in the other group have never been sued. They were balanced out in years in practice, procedures they performed, and so on. What Gladwell found was that the biggest difference between the sued group and the not-sued group was their tone of voice. Was it a dominating tone or a compassionate tone? Those with the compassionate tone fell into the not-sued group. Work on your tone. Are you coming off as condescending or dominating, or are you concerned and compassionate?

■ **Likeability:** The L in TLC stands for likeability. The components of likeability have been well documented in a book called *Influence*, by Dr. Robert Cialdini, who describes five components of likeability that I remember using the mnemonic "CASTA." C is compliments, A is attractive, S is similarity, T is team, and A is associations. So first, you should compliment patients on anything you like or that they did well. Here you can use a little flattery. When you compliment people, they just like it, even if they know it's flattery! It's not uncommon for me to say to a teenager whose mom brought him: "Oh, it's clear that your sister brought you in today." The mom finds that enjoyable, even if she knows I'm joking a little. Guess what? Moms love that. When I go to buy a suit, and they say, "You're very muscular in the shoulders, and you've clearly lost some weight since the last time you've been in here," those compliments go right to my head. Compliments are incredibly effective; use them wisely. When it comes to attractiveness, studies show that if you are physically attractive to another person, that person likes you more. Some of that is beyond your control, obviously, but you can still present yourself well and be neat and tidy. A lot of attractiveness simply boils down to smiling. When you're smiling and happy, that radiates to your patients. Next is similarity: I believe this is the biggest single trigger of likeability that you can immediately embrace. Whenever you find something in another person that you have in common, you need to highlight that similarity and talk about it. I believe that similarity is the key of human engagement and bedside manner. Similarity draws us to another; I believe it's a survival mechanism. Find something you have in common with a patient and talk about it. The next letter is T for team, meaning that when you go into a room, you need to let the patient know you're their advocate: I'm here for you. Yeah, I'm sorry you waited so long, I'm sorry that the nurse was a little bit rude, and I'm sorry about your past negative connotations with this facility. But I'm here for you now, I'm going to take care of you, and I'm your advocate. This goes over really well, especially if there is a significant time delay. I'll come in the room and say, "Boy, I'm sorry if you waited, I would be frustrated, too. I hate waiting in hospitals, so I'm sorry about that, but I'm here now and I'm going to take good care of you." About 80 percent of the patient's frustration melts right away. The last A is association. We like people who are associated with things that we like ourselves—this is a lot like similarity, but with more proof. If a patient likes fishing, and I talk a lot about my recent fishing trip, the patient has proof of my association with his own hobby.

■ **Compassion:** The C in TLC is compassion. How do you show compassion to your patients? My advice is that you shake everybody's hand when you walk into the room. It shows them that you care about them and that you respect them. Sit down as often as you can, which makes them think you're being more casual and not rushed. Actively listen to your patients rather than methodically running through your checklist of the HPI. Ask them questions that guide them to expand upon answers they gave, and nod your head. That's called back channeling. If they say something, acknowledge that you understand them: nod, squint your eyes, and say things like, "Got it, please go on." Always, always, always make comments about their time and about how you're sorry they waited so long. Even if they didn't wait long—say it anyways. Can't hurt.

Do not judge your patients. I repeat: do not judge your patients. A key ingredient to successful communication is not to accuse or place judgment on anyone. This is a very well-established principle in medicine—no patient is going to come into my emergency room and say, "Hey, can you give me judgment on how I'm living my life?"

A homeless guy who is homeless because of his disease, alcoholism, comes in smelling foul, hasn't taken a bath in months, reeks of liquor, and everything he owns is in a garbage bag. He's not coming in saying, "Hey John, what's your judgment of my life? Do you like it? Do you think I should keep living this way? Do you think that will be a good thing for me?" Absolutely not. He's here because he needs my help, and to the best of my ability, I need to help him without inflicting my own judgment. I need to *do my job*.

It's been shown that women who are obese have had more invasive gynecological cancer. For a long time, researchers thought that this correlation was due to the high estrogen levels produced by adipose tissue, to where any estrogen-dependent malignancy would become more aggressive. But eventually it was found that actually, obese women were less likely to get routine pelvic exams, because they were concerned about being judged by their clinicians.

That hurts me. The thought that a patient could fear—and worse, perceive—my thoughtless judgment and be prevented from opening up and receiving care hurts me, and it makes me feel that I need to be a better clinician and not let my attitude affect patients.

When I ask someone if they smoke, they're going to say, "Well, sometimes, but I cut down, I cut way down." Or, "No, I used to smoke, but I don't smoke anymore." Because they don't want my judgment or my crap about their lifestyle.

So it's very important that when I ask someone a question about their lifestyle, a question they may get defensive about, I have to say to them, "I'm not judging you, I just need to know so I can best take care of you." That has been a key component of my growth as a clinician and my ability to bridge communication gaps: decreasing the judgment that people perceive through how I frame questions. More importantly, it's what I truly believe and how I feel—that I don't have the right to judge any other person.

When you go out on rotations, you're going to start working from that paradigm immediately: that no patient wants your judgment, and that you need to constantly fight the urge to judge. You're there as a compassionate giver of medicine, a compassionate healthcare practitioner, and you must be very careful about being biased towards others, whether that means your patients, the nursing staff, your preceptors, or anyone else, for that matter.

Common Issues in Rotations

There are some issues that crop up for students during their clinical year, and my advice here is the same as it was for your didactic year. First and foremost, talk to your program—your advisor or the director—and be incredibly honest about where you are. If you're getting a divorce, if you or a loved one is dealing with a serious illness, or if you're going through some other kind of chaos or stress, you have to be very transparent. Even if you're dealing with an issue that is more self-induced, like drinking too much, you should still be transparent. PA school is such a natural system that you cannot be deceptive.

Many times, PA students have to deal with a lot of travel and staying in different housing while on rotations. Don't forget to use that travel time for your benefit, whether that means studying with your audio notes or catching up with old friends on the phone and recharging. Don't forget to take care of yourself, even if your schedule gets thrown off or you're living out of a hotel.

Burnout isn't as much of an issue in rotations as it is during the didactic year, because you're changing rotation sites so quickly. If you dislike a given rotation, it's not such a big deal, because you'll be gone in a couple of weeks.

But you very well may have other problems on your rotations. You could have a physician who is kind of abusing the PA and using the PA for free labor without really teaching—it happens. Another way that you could get into trouble on rotations is fraternization. This happens, too: preceptors fraternizing with students. You need to know that you have no obligation to do anything social with your preceptors whatsoever—if you want to go to an end-of-rotation celebration with a group, great, but it's certainly not a requirement. You may experience conflict with nursing staff. These are all issues that can crop up now and then, and again, I would just say that if you are facing a problem on a rotation, you need to be completely transparent with your advisor or program director; cut down the tree while it's a sapling instead of waiting for it to turn into an oak.

Some Final Words of Wisdom for Your Clinical Year . . .

"Ask questions! You have a personal teacher during this time—take advantage of it!"
—Maddie Windstein

"Do not auscultate through clothing. Do not palpate or examine the abdomen with the patient in the chair."
—Jocelyn Hook

"Clinical rotations will be the last time you can play the 'I can't do that because I'm just a student' card— so don't. Arrive early and stay late during clinical rotations; you learn the most when it's just you and your preceptor."
—Dr. Henry H. Heard

Chapter 4

Passing Your Boards: Preparing for the PANCE

"The PANCE has a national pass rate somewhere in the 90s. As such, it is not a difficult test in the traditional sense. It is a long, grueling test. Recognize you are preparing for it on day one of PA school, and you can't cram in the last month and expect to do well."
—Christopher Hanifin

You have a big test to take that a whole lot is riding on. Make no mistake about it, the PANCE is a comprehensive and difficult test. It's a primary care-based exam that's almost like an endurance event. The boards will make or break you. Passing your boards is the catch you have to make to win the game.

You'll probably never in your life take another test quite like this. The study techniques that got you through high school, college, and PA school will not get you through the boards. My hope is that you took my suggestion from chapter 3 and studied throughout your rotations. If you're reading this chapter and have not put much effort into studying for your boards up until now, you're going to have a steep mountain to climb. It's not insurmountable, but it is going to be tricky.

Studying for the boards, you need to strengthen your understanding of not just the natural system being tested—meaning, you will build upon your deep knowledge of medicine—but also the social system at play—meaning you will learn how you are being tested and what the test creators are looking for.

The Nature of the Test

First and foremost, you must understand that the boards are produced by the NCCPA—that is, academics who are deeply committed to PA education. These people do not want to trick you, but they do want to challenge you. They want to ensure that you have the knowledge base required to take excellent care of patients. Many of these test creators have specific fields of expertise, yet they may have been working in academia, outside of clinical practice, for a long time. They are not necessarily in tune with what is *common* in medicine.

The fact that the test creators are academics means that you may have some translational issues; the more casual terms you use in a clinical environment, like in your rotations, may be different from the more scientific terms employed in the test. Test creators are going to use textbook terms and may not use the abbreviations or shortcuts you are accustomed to. Rather than using the term "tripod position," they may say that a patient is leaning forward with arms extended and head tilted backwards. Rather than using the term "JVD," for jugular venous distention, they'll say a patient has distended neck veins.

Therefore, you have to become very familiar with academic terminology. If I say you supinate your wrist, what does that mean? What is a needle thoracotomy? This terminology can throw us off, because we would typically just say "a twisted wrist" or "a needle decompression." You need to know that laryngotracheitis is a fancy name for croup. If you don't study your medical terminology, you may completely miss a question, even though you have a really good knowledge base and could address the disease described by the question in a natural environment.

Understand that when you study for your boards, you need to think like a test writer. I am constantly asking students, "What would a test writer want you to know about this? How would a test writer ask a question about this topic?"

Knowing the breakdown of the test's topics is also important. If you go to the NCCPA website and look at their test blueprint, you can see which areas will be on the test—and furthermore, what percentage of the test is devoted to certain topics. So you can see that 48 percent of your boards will be comprised of four topics: cardiovascular, pulmonary, gastrointestinal, and musculoskeletal. This breakdown is very helpful and can help you to know how to allocate your study time proportionally to what areas will be tested.

However, here again you must be mindful of the difference between the academic and clinical perspectives. On the NCCPA website, you may note that infectious diseases make up only 3 percent of your boards. However, much of what you might consider to be infectious disease in clinical practice—for example, otitis media or meningitis—would fall under a different topic according to test creators. Otitis media would fall under the umbrella of ENT, and meningitis would be categorized as a neurological disease. So infectious diseases actually make up a fairly high portion of your boards, because as PAs, we care for patients with a very broad range of infectious diseases. This is important to remember.

Studying Smarter

I need to be very clear about this. Lots of people feel that answering a bunch of practice test questions is how they should study for their boards. I think that's a catastrophic mistake to make.

I believe test questions are an assessment tool, not a study tactic. What happens is that students practice answering questions, but when they get questions wrong, they simply try to understand and remember the *right* answer, rather than focusing on why they got the question wrong in the first place and really focusing their studying efforts there. The real studying begins once you identify *why* you got a given question wrong and then study not just what the question was asking, but all four of the foundational questions associated with the disease being asked about: pathophysiology, presentation, diagnosis, and plan.

Ideally, in order to help PA students prepare for the boards in the long term, I would have each student write academically sound questions on particular topics. I would want you to write questions that would pass peer review— questions that were medically well-founded, evidence-based, and aligned with what PAs need to know. Focus on those four questions; keep coming back to them over and over again. To really strengthen your knowledge of medicine, you should write all sorts of questions about a given topic, questions that address all four of those foundational questions. The deeper your knowledge is, the better able you'll be to write reasonable distractors—answers that sound like they could be correct but aren't—and test for exceptional presentations and patient-specific plans.

Students often think possessing tenuous knowledge is enough. If I ask you about cardiac risk factors, you can't waffle on it. You have to know those risk factors viscerally and rattle them off automatically: smoking, age, diabetes, cholesterol, hypertension, family history.

An alternative danger is when students spend time studying what they already know, reassuring themselves that they know a topic and proving to themselves they know it. Guess what? That makes you really good at the things you already know, and you don't put time in on the topics that will help you optimize your boards. This is like going to the gym and doing five-pound curls. Yes, you're doing work, yes, you're in the gym, but you're not getting stronger. Studying for your boards needs to be painful. It needs to be challenging, engaging, and taxing.

I stress this to you, folks: Do not allow yourself to be complacent. Push yourself. Pick up those heavier weights.

Tools to Utilize

Use review books that help you. Find one review book and go to work. I feel comfortable recommending three review books.

The first is *First Aid for the USMLE Step 2 CK*, 8th edition, by Le, Bhushan, and Skelley. The second is *PANCE Prep Pearls*, by Dwayne A. Williams. I've had the privilege of meeting Dwayne a number of times. I have tremendous respect for him, the work that he does, and the passion he has for getting PAs to succeed. Yet I can also say without bias, having taught CME4LIFE's board review course approximately fifty times, and having read a great number of review books, that I recommend this book highly. It's an excellent, comprehensive book that is a favorite among PAs.

Both of these are grade-A books. I have no bias to recommend them, other than having found them very helpful during my deep involvement in teaching board review.

Claire Babcock O'Connell's *A Comprehensive Review for the Certification and Recertification Examinations for Physician Assistants* is also a good and useful review book. That would be my third choice.

Use your PACKRAT results. There's a test out there called the Physician Assistant Clinical Knowledge Rating and Assessment Tool (PACKRAT) that was designed to mimic the PANCE. The PACKRAT is written by the Physician Assistant Education Association (PAEA) with the intention of providing students a gauge of where they stand before taking the boards. As 90 percent of PA schools administer the PACKRAT, most of you will take the PACKRAT during your senior year.

I know from working with PA schools that if your PACKRAT score is greater than 150, your odds of passing the PANCE are astronomically high. There's no reason why you should go into your boards without having a very clear understanding of where you stand. If you take the test and your score indicates you are on shaky ground, keep building your knowledge and working on the areas where you're weak in an in-depth, comprehensive way that focuses on the four questions of medicine.

Interpret your NCCPA pretest results. I recommend the NCCPA's pretests as a tool to guide your study focus. Each test is one hundred and twenty questions, and you are given one minute per question, so one hundred and twenty minutes.

Folks, all of the questions on these tests are old board questions, so you cannot take a pretest that's more aligned with your initial certification exam. I highly recommend you take this pretest. It will immediately give you a printout of where you're weak and where you're strong.

After the test, you can analyze your results and then get to work with the in-depth studying we've been describing. If you're not sure of where you need to study based on your results, please go to my website, contact me with your results, and I will respond to give you an overview of the areas you need to work on.

Those NCCPA pretests are an absolute goldmine. Use them to know where you stand and where you need to study.

> *"Take one NCCPA practice test two to three months out from your test date so you have an idea not only of which subjects you need to work on, but also what the actual questions look like. Take the other test two to three weeks out and reevaluate yourself and know where to hone in those last few weeks of studying."*
> —Maddie Windstein

Use CME4LIFE as a resource. My company, CME4LIFE, has created a range of tools that help organize and condense information and highlight patterns that will help you better understand the PANCE.

For the PANCE, you will need to have a thorough

understanding of similars: disease processes that present similarly but are different, such as epiglottitis versus croup, Crohn's versus ulcerative colitis, or a seborrheic keratosis versus actinic keratosis. These are all diseases that present similarly, but are very different. At CME4LIFE, we have simplified the process of studying these similars by coming up with a program called PA Prep JANUS.

You will also need to study demographics as they relate to disease processes. You need to know when certain disease processes hit people—at what age does a disease present? Test takers will not talk about a nineteen-year-old having a myocardial infarction, because that's extremely unlikely and uncommon. Test takers will not talk about a three-year-old having pyloric stenosis, because that happens in five-week-olds. To help students master demographics as they relate to disease processes, we came out with a product called PA Prep Timeline, which looks at what medical disease processes come up at what stages of life.

You need to pay attention to what populations are affected at disproportionate rates by certain disease processes. If a test question mentions race or vocation, it may be key to your understanding. For instance, if someone is a forest ranger, he is probably exposed to ticks. Farmers are exposed to sun and wind. If a test question mentions that a patient is African American, ask yourself what diseases and conditions occur more frequently among African Americans. You need to focus on most commons: questions that are framed in a way that asks the most common causes of certain disease states. What is the most common cause of microcytic anemia? You need to really focus on most commons.

I find that a lot of people do not know most commons. That's why we created a package of seven hundred and fifty flashcards for people to study that includes a lot of these types of questions. If you would like to access these flashcards free of charge, go ahead and download CME4LIFE's app called Quizlet.

We have programs and products at CME4LIFE that help you with all of these areas of focus, because we really try to serve you guys and simplify your studies.

A Word on Board Review Courses

There are many different board review courses out there, ranging anywhere from three to five days. Overall, I feel most PA students don't need a board review course. If you worked hard and diligently during your didactic year and on your rotations, then you probably don't even need a review course. If you're not sure if you need a review course, take the NCCPA pretest. It's pretty easy to do and to know where you stand.

When I got through the King's College PA program, I took the board review course at Yale University. It was very detailed, and I felt it confirmed a lot of the things that I knew already. I don't think it really allowed me to grow significantly. It was mostly overcrowded PowerPoint slides and people reading the slides aloud. I really struggle to say that the course was very beneficial.

Be careful about any board review course that just reads you slides. In too many of them, someone just puts an overburdened slide up in front of you and reads the words. If that is their method of teaching, then my advice is just to rent a hotel room, get with a couple of people, and read to each other. It'll save you time and money. It will be more efficient and more effective.

Many board review courses say they'll give you your money back if you fail, yet there are typically administrative fees that are nonrefundable, and some of the big organizations will actually subtract your food costs. If it's a $600 board review course, you may still end up paying $300, even if they refund your money, because of their administrative fee and your food cost.

If you have a traditional learning style, my advice is that no course manual is going to be as good as a good review book. I've already recommended the review books that I feel are your best bet.

My company, CME4LIFE, offers a board review course that I believe—albeit with maybe a little bit of bias— is the very best. It is nothing shy of extraordinary and transformative. Do not take my word for it. Look at the testimonials from people on YouTube and on our website to hear how enthusiastic people are about this course.

Not everyone may need our course, because some people learn very traditionally and can be adequately prepared from conventional lectures, readings, and memorization strategies. But a vast majority of students benefit tremendously from our board review course, because it is founded in active engagement learning. We know that people learn better when their brains are engaged, and we have had tremendous success with thousands of students based on the success rate and testimonials. So yes, I have a dog in this fight, but I truly believe ours is the best product out there right now.

Folks, if there's anything we can do here at CME4LIFE

to help you prepare for your boards, we will do it. We are passionately committed to this profession. Please check out our website and our YouTube channel, as we have about five hundred videos posted in which we're giving away a whole bunch of information for free.

Practical Guide to Testing

I've had the privilege of having some interactions with people on the PANCE committee. I absolutely respect the NCCPA and the integrity of the testing process. I do, however, feel very comfortable sharing the following tips. When it comes to studying for your PANCE, I call this our "study smart system."

Don't skip questions. When it comes to your boards, do not skip questions. If you skip a question, it is automatically wrong. There is absolutely no upside to skipping a question. Even if you plan to come back to it, don't skip it. Select an answer and note the question number so that you can return to it later and change your answer if necessary.

Stick and go. The next strategy is what I call stick and go, meaning if you don't know the answer, stick and go. Drop an answer down and move on. I would like you to think that on the PANCE there are going to be questions that are exploratory but mean nothing to your score. Tell yourself that they are testing some feature or concept that is simply outside the realm of what you are expected to know. I call these "Hail Mary questions." These are questions for which you have absolutely no idea what the right answers are, and so you just throw a Hail Mary pass and hope that someone miraculously catches it. Drop an answer and move right along.

The stick part is important because, again, there is absolutely no benefit to not putting down *some* answer, any answer, in hopes that it is correct. The go part is important because you do not want to get psyched out while you are taking the test. Do not mark it down to come back to if you are not ever going to know it. Do not worry a single extra second about that question. I teach people to try to have the psychology of a hockey goalie: If you get scored on, you shake it off and keep moving. You do not open yourself up to emotional sabotage.

The amount of information you can be tested about on the boards is so incredible and vast that no one can know it all. You are not expected to know it all. Stick and go.

Trust your gut. I love my gut. I cannot stress this enough. This has been talked about numerous times by advanced test writers. If you read a question and your gut is saying one thing, but your brain is saying another, go with your gut. I've done a lot of thinking, pondering, and studying about the subconscious and how the subconscious makes decisions. I know by now that the human brain can hijack itself and pull us into cognitive traps, and in fact this is a leading cause of medical errors.

When it comes to your boards, if your gut says one answer, but your brain says another answer, I would like you to go with your gut. Read the question through carefully, and be sure you're considering all possible aspects of the question—and then trust yourself.

Of course, you may want to test this strategy while studying and on pretests, just to see how often your gut is right. Yet I'm convinced that for almost everybody, the gut is dependable.

Dismiss answers that are new to you. I will not select an answer I've never heard of. When you read a base question, and you read an answer you have never heard before in your life, I would like you to exclude that answer. Assume it is a distractor—an incorrect response positioned to seem like a plausible response. It doesn't matter if it's a medicine, a test, or what have you—if something sounds foreign or you've never heard it worded that way, toss it.

Whether it's the name of a medicine or a particular diagnostic test, even if it sounds familiar to you, but you've never quite heard it worded that way, I'd like you to exclude that as a plausible distractor. As someone who has written test questions for colleges, I know that writing a question is not difficult. The real hard part is putting down plausible distractors that students consider marking correct. When it's impossible to come up with enough real distractors, we throw something down that seems legit and see if you'll bite. So again, trust yourself. If something seems new to you, don't take the bait.

Remember how often it's right to "do nothing." When you are asked about treatment plans, remember how often it's right to take the passive path. This is an absolutely huge part of selecting responses on your boards. As often as you can, do nothing. There are a great many disease processes out there for which the first step in treatment is lifestyle modifications. In essence, do nothing. Test creators do not want us, once we are PAs, to be too quick on the draw with our prescription pads.

What's the first step for treating hyperglycemia? Lifestyle modifications. What's the first step for hypertension? Lifestyle modifications. What's the first step for treating high cholesterol? Lifestyle modifications.

Realize also that there are a whole bunch of disease processes that we do nothing about, like a ganglion cyst. We simply observe and monitor. Fibroids? Observation. Benign prostate hyperplasia? Observation. If you see a response that in essence says "Do nothing," consider that response a strong contender for the correct answer.

Remember to protect the helpless. Likewise, remember that test creators want us, once we are PAs, to keep a watch out for those who are helpless: pediatric patients and geriatric patients. If you see a question about a strange disease presentation in a child or elderly patient, and you think, "Huh, that's strange, that could be cause for alarm," then give strong consideration to any response indicating you should report what you see.

What to Expect

Understand that when you show up on test day, it's an incredibly sterile environment. You walk in with your two forms of ID, and you will have to have been registered for the test with the exact name that is on your ID, or they will bounce you and not allow you to take the test. They will take your picture, and you'll have a palm print that they put on file so they can identify you specifically.

You'll walk back into a room where the security is tighter than at the airport. Everything that you do during testing is going to be video and audio recorded. You'll have structured breaks. It can be quite intimidating.

During the test, there are a couple of things that are available to you. One is a drop-down menu of normal lab values. That's helpful if you're looking for an uncommon lab, but you should go into your boards understanding the top eighteen most common labs and their values. Again, you can find a resource for this information on CME4LIFE's website.

You also will have a sheet of paper or a dry-erase board that you can write on, but you cannot write on it until the test begins. My advice is that as soon as you begin, you immediately write down all the mnemonics and memory aides you've memorized so that they are available to you throughout the test and you don't need to interrupt your momentum. Again, we have a sheet of suggested mnemonics available on our website for a wide range of topics.

It normally takes about two weeks for you to get your results back, and you'll usually get your results on a Thursday morning.

Managing Boards Anxiety

Boards anxiety could be an entire chapter in itself. You feel that your entire future hinges on this test, and of course you are putting a lot of pressure on yourself. Understand that this is indeed just a test. This test does not determine your self-worth, and it doesn't determine anything about what kind of long-term practitioner you're going to be.

It is a big test, but trust that you're going to be fine.

For the very small percentage of people who fail their boards the first time, 97 percent pass it the second time. Hopefully you have been studying throughout your entire journey and are feeling prepared. If you are wracked with anxiety, particularly to the extent that it is making you ill or you feel it is going to handicap your test taking ability, you need to address it. If you feel anxiety is really a large component of you taking the boards, then that needs to be resolved before you go into the test.

Use methods that you know work for you. Try to be optimistic, take care of your body, and seek out the support of friends and loved ones. Seek medical help if need be. You can also feel free to contact me directly through my website, and I will discuss your particular situation with you and recommend some strategies that may help you to be more confident and proactive. I respond to 100 percent of the people who reach out to me.

My number one rule is this: No cramming the day before your boards. A full day before your boards, a full twenty-four hours before you take the test, you are done. You are not allowed to study anymore. I command you to close your books and put away your notes. You need to be in the right mindset, feeling calm and prepared. If you are scrambling and feeling like there are still things you don't know, that is going to be toxic to your mindset. You can't start getting the yips. Get relaxed. Get confident. Get enough sleep; drink enough water.

I am very serious about this. Put away your notes. This day before your boards must be devoted to taking great pride in yourself and meditating on your wonderful accomplishments. I want you to walk into your boards with a positive mental attitude and laser focus.

Some Final Words of Wisdom for Your Board Prep . . .

"Regarding the PANCE exam, there should not really be any surprises—either you're ready or you're not. The NCCPA has practice exams available, and there are plenty of other third-party books and websites that also offer practice exams. Use these practice exams to gauge your knowledge and areas of deficiency. Study everything, but especially the content areas that you are deficient in. Repeat this process until you are consistently doing well on the practice exams, and then you can confidently know that you are ready for the real thing."
—Gerald Weniger

"How to pass the boards? Study, of course. If you are lucky, your program will provide a board review course, like CME4LIFE."
—Deborah Summers

"I always warn students taking the PANCE that it is very difficult to get a sense of how well you are doing on the test while you are taking it. In PA school you can sit down for a test and think, 'I am knocking this one out of the park!' It is very common for even high-performing, high-scoring students to feel very uncomfortable while taking the PANCE. Don't let it get into your head."
—Christopher Hanifin

Chapter 5

Life After PA School

As someone who's studied leadership and growth, and as someone who has experienced learning struggles and has had a bunch of bumps in the road, I know that PA school can be a very challenging journey. My hope is that my experience and advice help you to get the most out of PA school, create a fertile garden within you to absorb and nurture medical knowledge, and grow into a clinician who will have the capacity to help hundreds of thousands of patients during your time in medicine.

I hope that as you move into your professional career, you take great pride in your work and bring honor to the PA field.

Getting a Job

Don't just look for a job—look for the *right* job.
Particularly in the Northeast, where there are a lot of PA schools, a job that opens to new PA school graduates may have forty or fifty applicants. Too many students go to an interview desperate to have the job; they're like Oliver Twist begging for more. Remember, you don't just want to find a job—you want to find the *right* job.

When a physician gets out of medical school, they still don't know everything, and they have to work as a resident for three years. The same is essentially true for you—basically, you will be a resident physician, meaning you will still be in training, and nobody will expect you to have all the answers. Yes, you will have some degree of knowledge and understanding from the classroom and from your clinical rotations, but being a PA student is very different than being a working PA.

Your first job has got to be for the learning. This is so important. If on your first job, you are making $100,000 per year but are poorly supervised and are not growing as a provider, that is nowhere near as desirable as being the PA who gets out and makes $60,000 but sees a boatload of patients and is very well-supervised and is thoroughly trained.

Look at your goals. Where do you want to go? Where do you want to be in five years? Where do you want to be in ten years? Is a job going to get you the clinical knowledge and other opportunities to get there?

I think some students feel that when they graduate, the worst-case scenario is not to have a job, but that is not the worst-case scenario. The worst-case scenario is finding yourself in a job that is a bad fit, leads you to form bad habits, or doesn't offer any supervision, to where you do things wrong and harm patients.

Keep fantastic records. Any time you have an official piece of paperwork—for example, your official license to practice—put it into three different and distinct files: a file for master copies, a file for physical copies, and a file for digital copies. Have all of your official documents in triplicate. So as soon as you get your state license, you have it in one safe place, you make a photocopy of it, and you scan it and put it in your computer file. A real bane of

my PA career has been applying for jobs and not having
a single, centralized location for all of my paperwork.
I always had to spend a day tracking down paperwork.
If right from day one you maintain very well-organized
systems, it will pay off in dividends as you grow.

Keep your CV current and amazing. Keeping your
CV constantly updated is a great idea. Many programs
offer resources to help you with your CV, and I definitely
recommend taking advantage of any resources available
to you.

I'll give you two unique pieces of advice when it
comes to your CV. First, as you get your letters of reference,
take snippets from those and include them beside the
corresponding jobs or experience, almost like taglines,
with attributions for who said these great things about you.
This way, when an interviewer is looking down at your CV,
they're also seeing attention-getting endorsements: "Super
hardworking," "Nurses loved him," "A joy to be around."
I love this—it's one of the most powerful resume tricks
I ever saw. I couldn't read this guy's resume without saying,
"Holy cow, this guy is spectacular."

My second piece of CV advice for you is that at the
bottom, you have to include what I call an opener—some
achievement, award, or goal that an interviewer will not be
able to resist asking you about. This should be something
lighthearted and something you will be able to speak
engagingly about. On my CV, I include that I've won the
award for Greatest Hockey Dad of the Year for fifteen years
running. So the fact that I am an incredibly passionate
hockey dad comes up in every interview. Pick something
unique about yourself, something that stands out. I advised

one of my students to do this, and she told me she had no
idea what kind of opener she could include on her CV. We
brainstormed on it, and finally she goes, "Well, one time
I won second place in a wakeboarding competition." I said,
"Whoa, what is that?" and she went into this description of
wakeboarding. I told her that was *it*. That had to go on her
resume—it was interesting and I wanted to talk to her about
it. So she put it on her resume, and after her first interview
she couldn't call me fast enough. "Oh my gosh," she said,
"that is *exactly* what they opened with—they asked me,
'What is wakeboarding?'" Give yourself a good, intriguing
opener that will set the tone for the interview and allow your
interviewer to see you in a more personal way.

Do some recon. When you're trying to get your first job—
or later jobs, for that matter—you can use the strategy of
enlisting the help of insiders. If you are going to go interview
with a gastroenterology group and have scheduled an
interview with a gastroenterologist, my advice is to call
the practice and ask to speak to the PA who is on. When
the PA gets on the phone, you say, "Hey, I am hoping you
can help me. I am coming in to interview with your group,
and I sure would like to know a little more about the group
before the interview. Do you have five minutes to talk to
me?" The PA who is taking the phone call is going to say
yes, not only because you've worded your request so
politely, but also because there is a reasonable chance
they are going to be working with you, and they want to get
on your good side and have a good relationship. If the call
goes well, as soon as that PA sees the gastroenterologist,
they are going to say, "Hey, that PA you're interviewing
tomorrow called, and I talked to her for ten minutes—I like

this one." You are going to look like a shooting star, a really proactive person, and that is just win-win good stuff.

Ace your interview. In your interview, I encourage you to use the phrase "mutual good fit." You want to ensure that you would be happy in a job and the job would be happy with you. Not that you should come in guns blazing, demanding the world, because you are still just a student, and you need to be respectful. But it is really important to investigate the company culture. Most medical practices and hospitals don't articulate their cultures, per se, the way many businesses do when they verbalize their core values. Try to gather what evidence you can. Have they trained many PAs before? How many PAs have they trained, and how long have those PAs been with the company or the business or the hospital? Also, try to get a read on what your schedule would be like. If you'd be making $100,000 but working eighty-hour weeks, that is not actually so great. If you are able to come and shadow the PA on duty, that is a great way to set yourself far and away above the other applicants.

Your First Job: Learn from John the Jester

I was fired from my first job, and it really wasn't an issue of my capability; it was a human engagement issue. I didn't know how to engage with physicians or with the nursing staff. Eventually, they pulled me into the office and asked me to find a new job. It was extremely hard. With time and distance, I understood the mistakes I had made back when I was John the Jester.

I found there are four major strategies that will help you engage your colleagues at a very high level, and I recommend you try to employ them constantly, as I do.

Wear glasses of sincere appreciation. In my first job, I was not very appreciative. I am happy to say that now I wear glasses of sincere appreciation. These glasses, when I put them on, allow me to see those around me in such a way that I sincerely respect and appreciate them, and I work hard to communicate to them what I see. But more importantly, I work hard to realize that everybody's got their own story. Everybody's got good parts of them and bad parts of them.

When I put these glasses on, I see people by their potential—just as when you see a bird on a fence, you assume it can fly. That's also how we should see people: What you actually see is how people are engaging in their daily routines, but you should always strive to see them based on their capacity to be extraordinary creatures of a loving creator. Try to see in everyone the potential to fly.

Understand something, folks, this is not flattery. Flattery is counterfeit, and it's manipulative, and it's very selfish. Flattery is telling people things they want to know about themselves so that they like you better. I'm talking about recognizing the beauty and authenticity of each human being, and I'm talking about developing your ability to recognize those things. If you indeed are able to see beauty and authenticity in someone, the way you treat that person will reflect what you see, and that person will be able to live up to that potential. If you are working with a very grouchy nurse, and you can tell that the nurse has a certain talent, then you can point that out and honor her specific talent. I guarantee you that the nurse will be less grouchy towards you, because the nurse feels seen and understood and feels gratified when she can realize her potential.

Avoid complaining and be positive. There's a real negative side to human nature, and that is that it's easy to be a whiner, a pisser, and a moaner. Some people just get by in life by complaining and whining all the time, and it really sucks the life out of those around them. I certainly dabbled in this behavior during my first job, complaining about all sorts of things that didn't really matter.

When I go into PA schools, I have the whole class take their pointer fingers and put them in the air. I say, "On the count of three, I want you to point to the person in the class who's the biggest whiner, pisser, and moaner."

There's always this nervous crescendo of laughter as I start counting to three. Everybody's afraid of an uncomfortable situation—pointing to someone or being pointed at. I always stop the exercise and ask, "Would anybody be pointing to you?"

I make it very clear that if people would point to you and you're good with that, then I don't want to work with you. Know that you may have a fine role in the operating room, but not in a position where you're engaging with patients or clinicians very much.

Are you one of those people who whine, piss, and moan all the time? If so, are you good with that? Does that behavior let you be who you want to be and realize your full potential?

Avoid giving orders and ask for help. When I first became a PA, I took a Marine Corps attitude into the emergency room. I felt that my rank as a PA gave me authority over others, and I was drastically wrong. My paradigm was that I was the boss and people were going to do what I told them to do. This attitude was toxic, and it ultimately led to my being fired from my first job. You want to always be asking: How do I best serve patients? How do I best serve my supervising doc? How do I best serve the team?

Now that I have my mind-set right, I no longer tell anybody to do anything. I ask for their help. I no longer say, "Go get me vital signs." I ask, "Can you do me a favor and get orthostatic vital signs?" Or, "Can you do me a favor and get visual acuity?" Clearly in the emergency room, I give orders when there's an emergency—but the fact is that 99.8 percent of the time, that type of implementation of orders is not necessary. You need to establish your credibility and respect during that 99.8 percent of the time so that during the 0.2 percent of the time when critically ill patients come in, you can be commanding in an effective, positive way.

Avoid judgment and preserve others' dignity.

Understand that we all have our delusions, and we all rationalize. Even most criminals in jail don't think they're bad people. Everybody defends their own ego, and they do it aggressively at times, especially if there's a delusion involved.

As clinicians, we shouldn't challenge anybody's ego, and it's not our job to help people uncover their delusions. I work very hard to preserve egos in everyone I deal with. I don't tell anybody they're wrong, I just talk from my own experiences, and I try to guide them. I work very hard not to judge my patients, my nursing staff, or the docs I work with.

As a PA, you're going to see all kinds of personalities. You will have people who have a high degree of self-awareness and love for their profession, and you will also have the opposite—people who are struggling with interpersonal skills or ego and often take this out on patients and students. Do your best to preserve other people's egos, and try not to judge them, because you don't know their situation. If you think someone is doing something wrong, don't make it your business unless you absolutely have to, and even then just make it clear that you are seeking clarification.

It is very important to keep your mouth shut and not have an opinion about a lot of things. If someone is trying to recruit you to have an opinion, do your best just to watch, listen, take things in, and avoid being dragged into clashes. It is mature and acceptable to say, "You know, I don't have much of an opinion on that. I never really thought of that, and I just don't have much of an opinion."

If a provider or nurse talks in a derogatory way about a patient, never ever feed into that. That becomes toxic very quickly. Be polite and respectful, and treat the nurses incredibly well as fellow team players. That means answering the phones and cleaning up your own messes. It means if a patient needs a boost, you go give a boost. If a patient needs a rectal temp, go help the nurse hold the patient. If you're a team player, that gets around quickly.

Your Life as a PA

When you become a PA, you may experience a culture shift. In some ways, you are moving from adolescence to adulthood, and depending on your background, you may also experience a shift in socioeconomic position. You're going to be making good money and spending the majority of your time with working professionals, and while hopefully you feel great about where you are, it's possible you'll feel a little bit disoriented. From the get-go, do your best to be responsible. Put 10 percent of all your money into a retirement account straightaway.

I encourage you to always set goals, and this has to be pen to paper. The more detailed your goals are, the better. This is important: when you tell your subconscious what to focus on, destiny will align itself with what you've written down. Think about where you want to be one, three, five years from now, think about the kind of medicine you want to be practicing, think about the amount of money that you want to make, and think about what hobbies and fulfillment you want to pursue outside of your career.

Please continue learning—PAs should all be lifelong learners. Identify your deficiencies and take very active steps to remedy them. You have to actively and mindfully look at your practice and see where are you weak. Exercise that metacognition we've been talking about. I think it is very poor PA whose doc has to finally come to them and say, "You suck at EKG's, and you need to fix this." It is a very strong PA who goes to their doc and says, "I am realizing I have a deficit here, and I want to fix it. Here is my plan to fix it. What do you think of this? Is it a good plan?" Choose educational conferences that will help to fill your gaps.

I will leave you with this: Please take excellent, wonderful care of your patients. When you put on your jacket as PA and you begin to practice medicine, you absolutely surrender your right to judge patients' lifestyles. You will be caring for people who have made different life choices than you or who come from very different backgrounds than you, people whose lives you do not know or understand. Release your ego and your pride. Remember that your practice of medicine is not for you or about you. Remember that medicine is about perception, and patients need to perceive that you support them, and they need to like and respect you.

I had the opportunity, in 2015, to speak with Ken Ferrell, the first PA who graduated from the first PA program, at Duke University. I had the pleasure of meeting and interviewing him in front of a thousand PAs during a conference at the North Carolina Academy of Physician Assistants. I said, "Ken, as the first PA in the world, what is one thing you would want all these PAs to know?"

Ken thought for a moment and quoted Theodore Roosevelt, saying, "Nobody cares how much you know until they know how much you care." The most struggling patients need your compassion the most. While it is easy to love and extend generosity to a very likable patient, it takes a person of real character and integrity to be respectful to someone on the other side of the coin.

Love your patients. Care for your patients. I hope you have a fulfilling, rich, and wonderful career.

About the Author

John Bielinski, Jr. holds a master of science in emergency and family medicine and actively works as a PA in Western New York.

Growing up, John struggled in school, was labeled a "difficult learner," and was put in classes for students with special needs. He felt inadequate and stupid based on his inability to thrive using traditional learning methods.

After high school, feeling unprepared for college, John joined the United States Marine Corps and was soon deployed to Operation Desert Storm. John's job was to quickly and accurately recognize armored vehicles in order to identify the enemy. Any mistake could mean the loss of American lives. *John had to learn quickly and effectively.* The military provided John with a unique learning tool—flashcards. One side of each card had a picture of the vehicle; the other side listed identifying features. John found himself learning quickly, and he remembered what he'd learned. This strategy would serve as the basis for John's future teaching methods, designed to reach students of diverse learning styles.

After returning from duty, John completed his undergraduate degree at the University of Buffalo, went to PA school at King's College, and moved into clinical practice. He also developed a passion for teaching, serving as an instructor for ten years at two different PA schools in Buffalo, New York. Throughout his education and career, John developed and refined consistent, high-caliber, reproducible systems not only for teaching and learning, but also for assessing and treating patients.

John founded CME4LIFE, a continuing medical education company, after growing frustrated by conferences and learning tools that failed to engage learners. His unique approach—"Active Engagement Learning"—weaves together storytelling, song and dance, memorable mnemonics, audience participation, and an emphasis on critical thinking, making CME4LIFE's products more engaging and effective than anything else out there.

John feels strongly that God has given him the gift of teaching to share with passionate medical providers.

About CME4LIFE

CME4LIFE (https://cme4life.com) is committed to helping people become better, more effective medical providers. With our innovative, engaging content—products, conferences, and many free resources—continued medical education comes alive and helps people learn better, faster, and with higher retention. We understand that people learn differently and that traditional teaching methods aren't for everyone—which is why we teach in ways that guide people not to memorize the material, but to truly *understand* it.

Approved by the AAPA, we're focused on high-end medicine taught simply. We're dedicated to making difficult material easy to learn and recall. We provide a convenient way to earn CME credits. Our company was created for clinicians, by a clinician. Our team is passionate, personalized, and driven to help people reach their career goals.

Products

CME4LIFE offers a variety of DVDs, textbooks, audio files, and other study tools that cover a range of medical topics. These materials are fun, engaging, and impactful—meaning you'll actually remember the content and enjoy learning it!

PA Board Review CME

- *Demystifying the PA Boards* – 16-DVD series
- *PA Prep Catapult* – audio/text PA study kit
- *PANCE/PANRE PA Prep Essentials Flashcards*
- *Elemental Medicine* by John Bielinski, Jr., MS, PA-C – textbook
- *PA Prep Medical Triads* – text/audio
- *PANCE Prep Pearls* – textbook
- PANCE Private Tutoring Options Available – limited basis – contact CME4LIFE for details

Clinical Medicine CME

- *Demystifying Acute Care Medicine* – DVD series
- *Conquering Cardiology* – DVD series
- *Black Belt ECG* – DVD series
- *Secrets of Urgent Care* – DVD series
- *Advanced Emergency Medicine* – DVD series
- *Hospitalist Medicine* – DVD series

Self-Assessment CME

- Acute Care, Orthopedic, or General Medicine/ Primary Care – live conference and workbook

Performance Improvement CME

- Medical Malpractice or Patient Satisfaction – DVD and workbook

CPSIA information can be obtained
at www.ICGtesting.com
Printed in the USA
BVHW070038090519
547814BV00002B/169/P